Intermittent Fasting for Women

Strategy Guide for Beginners

SARAH TAYLOR

Text Copyright © Sarah Tylor

All rights reserved. No part of this guide may be reproduced in any form without the written permission from the publisher, except in case of brief quotations in critical articles or reviews.

Legal Disclaimer

The information contained in this guidebook is not designed to replace or take the place of any form of medical advice or independent medical, financial, legal, or other professional services, as may be necessary. The content provided is strictly meant for educational and entertainment use only.

The information available in this guide has been compiled from reliable sources and is accurate to the best of the Author's knowledge and belief. However, the Author cannot guarantee the accuracy and validity, and cannot be held liable for any errors or omissions. Further, modifications will be periodically made to this book as and when the Author deems fit.

Upon using the contents and information included in this book, you agree to hold the Author and affiliated parties harmless from and against any damages, expenses, and costs, including any legal fees potentially resulting from the implementation of any of the information contained in this book. This disclaimer applies to any loss, harm or injury caused due to the use and application, whether directly or indirectly, of any advice presented, whether for breach of contract, criminal intent, tort, personal injury, negligence, or under any other course of action.

You consent to accept all risks of using the information given inside this book.

You also agree that by continuing to read this book, where appropriate and necessary, you shall consult a professional (including but not limited to your doctor, attorney, or financial advisor or such other consultant as needed) before using any of the suggested remedies, techniques, or information in this book.

Introduction

Are you tired of being bombarded by countless infomercials about new diets that only give partial results? I'm pretty sure you've heard about the ketogenic diet, paleo diet, vegan diet, and even the raw food diet. Now, I'm not criticizing or taking jabs at any of these, and I do genuinely believe in most cases, these diets do work effectively to a certain degree.

But you see there lies an inherent problem with all these so-called "diets." People tend to go on them and start seeing some results in the beginning. However, before they know it, they start gaining back those unwanted pounds simply because they couldn't uphold their regimen. To add insult to injury, a lot of these diets tend to be quite expensive, and thus, an average working person fails to afford them.

Well, I'm here to tell you that Intermittent Fasting (IF) won't cost you any more than what you are already spending. This diet, in particular, is designed to help you burn unwanted body fat fast and sculpt your ideal physique in conjunction to exercise.

Intermittent Fasting has been taking the health and fitness world by storm lately. All over the world, people following all kinds of diets and all kinds of lifestyles are weaving fasting windows into their daily lives to help improve their physical and mental health as well as their wellness progression.

This book has been specifically created for women interested in Intermittent Fasting as a wellness tool that assists them in achieving their personal health goals. The following chapters will not only discuss the basics of IF as a means of weight loss and health enhancement, but they will also cover topics that are specific to women health.

By the end of the guide, you will feel more comfortable about the concept of Intermittent Fasting, and all that defines it. This will enable you to take your first steps with confidence and take advantage of all the benefits the program has to offer. Even though females need to take greater care when preparing their IF routines than men, there is an abundance of positive health benefits women can gain from the right fasting schedule.

Keep this book by your side throughout your IF journey. When questions arise, or changes need to be made to your personal fasting routine, this book will be the quick reference guide that will help you to maximize the benefits or eliminate any adverse effects.

Packed with useful and valuable information from cover to cover, Intermittent Fasting for Women is a robust planning and preparation tool for women interested in starting their first Intermittent Fasting plan. The main goal of this guide is to help you reach your best physical, mental, and emotional health with a strong and reliable personalized IF program.

You probably decided to buy this book because you want to become a better version of yourself! Well, the good news is you have made the best decision. Your life will be transformed once you start implementing the strategies I discuss in this book.

Yes, you read it right, this book is going to change your life! I know you just started reading, but I'm serious! My book is designed to impact your life in the most positive way possible from a holistic standpoint.

However, before I start with the basics of Intermittent Fasting, we need to get your mindset right! Something that is often ignored within the health and fitness industry is having a good sense of self-awareness before starting any diet. As mentioned previously, the fundamental issue with all diets is that people cannot uphold or continue with their diet routines.

But why? It is because people treat diets like prescription drugs! Once results are derived and an outcome is finalized, people tend to go back to their old ways of living and relegate their newfound diet fad to the back burner.

In short, people consider diet as a short term fix, and this is the root of all disappointments. True transformation can only take place from the inside out and when you become self-aware, changing the way you eat is not a matter of going on a short term diet, but a total lifestyle change!

That's right. You need to transform your lifestyle or modify it in order to achieve long term sustainable results! You need to incorporate Intermittent Fasting as a part of your daily living, and to do this, you must shift your mindset to "IF is not a prescription drug."

Within the past few years, the concept of Intermittent Fasting has started to trend heavily, impacting anyone interested in dieting and healthy living. Its origins, however, are much more ancient than most of us would ever imagine. In the following chapter, you'll be introduced to the long history of Intermittent Fasting so that you can better understand how that trajectory leads to today. By the end of the section, you will feel confident that you know where the tradition comes from, as well as what it has to do with you—reading this book in this very moment.

Table of Contents

Intermittent _____ 15

Fasting _____ 15

   What Is Intermittent Fasting? _____ 16

   Origins: Where Did Intermittent Fasting Come From? _____ 20

      Intermittent Fasting Tip: Apple Cider Vinegar _ 24

   What Happens to the Food You Eat? _____ 25

      Intermittent Fasting Tip: Fasting Is Habit & Determination, Not A Miracle Cure _____ 27

   The Science of Intermittent Fasting: How Does It Work? _____ 28

   Why Should You Practice Intermittent Fasting? _ 30

   What are the Disadvantages of Intermittent Fasting? _____ 31

Chapter 2 _____ 34

Intermittent Fasting for Women _____ 34

   Intermittent Fasting & The Female Form _____ 35

How Does Intermittent Fasting Benefit Women? 37

How Is Intermittent Fasting Riskier for Women? 40

Step One: Making A Plan That Will Get Results ___ 41

    Asking the Right Questions _____ 42

    Gather All the Information You Can _____ 43

    Determine Your Motivation & Set Realistic Goals _____ 44

    Getting Your Body Accustomed To Fasting ___ 46

    Intermittent Fasting Tip: The Best First Step Is the Baby Step _____ 47

    Step Two: Choosing A Realistic Intermittent Fasting Plan _____ 48

Chapter 3 _____ 50

Intermittent Fasting: Benefits, Side Effects & Precautions _____ 50

    Aging Process _____ 52

    Lowered Cardiovascular Risk _____ 53

    Intermittent Fasting For Cancer Prevention ____ 54

- Brain Power and Aging _____ 55
- Calorie Independent Effect _____ 56
- Side Effects of Intermittent Fasting _____ 57
- Precautions to Take _____ 58
  - Who Should Avoid Intermittent Fasting? _____ 58
  - Who Needs To Be Cautious? _____ 60

Chapter 4 _____ 61

Autophagy Revolution _____ 61
- The Origin of Autophagy _____ 63
- The Benefits of Autophagy _____ 64
- The Process of Autophagy _____ 66
  - Autophagy Vs. Apoptosis _____ 67
  - How to Induce Autophagy? _____ 68
  - Dry Fasting & Water Fasting _____ 74
  - Intermittent Fasting, Autophagy & Anti-Aging – The Intersection _____ 77

Chapter 5 _____ 79

- 8 Types of Intermittent Fasting Diets 79
  - The 16/8 Method: A Popular Choice 82
  - An Ideal Option for Women of All Ages: The 5/2 Intermittent Fasting Plan 85
  - Crescendo Fasting 88
  - Eat Stop Eat 91
  - Alternate Day Fasting 94
  - The Warrior Method 97
  - Fat Fasting 100
  - Fasting Mimicking Diet 106
- Intermittent Fasting to Lose Weight 110
  - Step Three: Fit Bodies Are Made In The Kitchen _ 112
    - Stock Your Kitchen To Support An Intermittent Fasting Routine 113
    - Example Meal Plan For Weight Loss With Intermittent Fasting 116
  - Step Four: Be Prepared To Exercise Before You Jump Right In! 121

Exercising With Intermittent Fasting _____ 121

Get A Professional Opinion To Guarantee Health & Safety _____ 125

Intermittent Fasting Tip: Keep A Record Of Your Personal Experience _____ 126

Step Five: Schedule Your First Fasting Plan _____ 128

Plan Out More Than Just One Week At A Time 129

Choosing The Best Day To Start A New Intermittent Fasting Routine _____ 130

What To Expect In The First Week On A New Intermittent Fasting Schedule _____ 131

Intermittent Fasting Tip: Drink More Water Than Before _____ 133

Step Six: Know How To Continue Your Fast _____ 134

Intermittent Fasting in Our Life _____ 138

Intermittent Fasting &How It Affects Your Hormones _____ 141

Intermittent Fasting & Paleo Diet _____ 143

Intermittent Fasting & Vegan Diet _____ 150

Intermittent Fasting & Keto Diet _____ 161

Conclusion _____ 169

   An Important Warning: _____ 172

   Tips To Succeed At Intermittent Fasting _____ 173

   Busting Common Intermittent Fasting Myths ___ 178

   Questions About Intermittent Fasting _____ 180

   To Summarize Everything _____ 186

Resources Page _____ 189

Chapter 1

Intermittent Fasting

What Is Intermittent Fasting?

Intermittent Fasting (IF) is no diet, but a dietary pattern. In simplest terms, it is consciously deciding to skip certain meals. Fasting and then eating deliberately, IF means eating the calories for a specific time of the day and choosing not to eat food outside of that particular time.

Now, you may be thinking, "Okay, by skipping a meal, I end up eating less than normal, and therefore, I'm going to lose weight, right?" Well, that is partially true. Yes, by eliminating a meal, you can consume MORE food during your other meals and at the same time consume fewer calories (which is vital for losing weight). However, since it is known that not all calories are the same, the meal schedule can also influence the way your body reacts.

There are several methods of Intermittent Fasting. The most popular are:

- Skip two meals in one day, making it a total of 24 hours of fasting. For example, eat at a normal time (ending dinner at 8 pm) and then do not eat again until 8 pm the next day.
- The 16/8 mode: It is known as the "Leangains" approach. As per this method, you can eat for 8 hours, and then you have to fast

for 16. The normal fasting time includes sleep and a few extra hours. You can skip breakfast, for instance, and make the first meal at noon and continue beating until 8.

- Diet 5: 2: The idea is that during two days of the week, you lessen your calorie intake to 500-600 calories a day. The days do not have to be consecutive. The additional five days you can eat whatever you want.

Eat, stop, and eat: This kind of Intermittent Fasting substitutes fasting days with days of eating. You eat what you need for 24 hours, and then you take a total lunch intermission the next day. You have to imitate this pattern like twice a week. Drinks without calories are allowed.

Your Hormonal Balance Also Changes

Practicing IF does much more than restrict caloric intake. It also changes the body's hormones so that they can make better use of your fat reserves. The following changes occur:

- Intermittent Fasting improves **insulin sensitivity** in combination with exercise. This is very relevant for people who have weight problems because low insulin levels are related to better fat burning.

- The opposite case is **insulin resistance**. Some studies have shown that an increase in weight can interfere with insulin's ability to lower blood sugar levels, resulting in more insulin. This favors the storage of fat.
- The secretion of the Human Growth Hormone (HGH) or the "fitness hormone" increases, accelerating the synthesis of protein and making fat available as an energy source. This means, in a nutshell, that you burn fat and build muscles more quickly. That's why growth hormone is taken in significant quantities by bodybuilders as a doping agent.

Also, according to research, fasting activates autophagy, which helps the body's regeneration process by repairing or eliminating damaged cells.

Should You Follow the "Eat 6 Small Meals a Day" Theory?

When you consume food, your body has to burn extra calories to process that food. The theory "Eat 6 Small Meals A Day" states that if you eat small meals all day long, your body is always burning calories and your metabolism is working at its optimum capacity.

Well, that's not true. If you eat 2,000 calories spread throughout the day or 2,000 calories in a short amount of time, your body will still burn the same amount of calories when processing food. Therefore, "keep your metabolism working at its optimum capacity by always eating" sounds good in principle, but reality says otherwise.

When you eat smaller meals, you are less likely to overeat during regular meals. This is especially true in the case of people who struggle with portion control or do not know how much food they should eat actually to benefit from it.

But, once you educate yourself and take control of your diet by practicing Intermittent Fasting, eating six times a day is prohibitive, and it requires a lot of effort. Also, because you are eating six small meals, you will probably never feel "full," and there is a chance that you will consume MORE calories in each snack. Due to this specific reason, the "six meals a day" is not recommended for most people.

You Will Lose Weight If You Do It Well

If you want to lose weight, you will have to limit your calorie intake. Some researchers have found that Intermittent Fasting if done correctly, can be useful both to prevent Type 2 diabetes and to reduce calories. It also helps the body to learn how to process the food absorbed during the period of eating more efficiently.

Other studies have found that a mixture of the 16/8 method and strength training can reduce more fat than energy training alone. This also means that IF is expressly effective when you combine it with regular workouts.

However, Intermittent Fasting is not significantly beneficial for pregnant or lactating women or people who have high blood pressure. So, you should consult your doctor before changing your eating habits.

Origins: Where Did Intermittent Fasting Come From?

Fasting has been a natural part of life in one form or another since the origins of humankind. At its most basic level, fasting is a tool developed by early humans to survive during extended periods without food such as deep winter, when many animals are in hibernation, or after natural disasters such as plagues or floods, when crops were unexpectedly destroyed

Instead of just giving in to starvation or going straight to uprooting their community in search of more bountiful lands, they learned to restrict their calorie intake and ration their food to only consume enough to survive and make their reserves last, until conditions improved.

But in modern times, apart from survival, in countries and cultures across the planet, fasting is most commonly associated with religious practices, devotion, and ceremony. Long-standing religions with the most ancient roots are known to incorporate some form of fasting into their beliefs.

Muslims fast during the holy month of Ramadan as a way of displaying their devotion to their faith. This form of fasting is more absolute than those used for medical and dieting purposes. During the 12-hour daily fasting window (sunrise to sunset), in addition to food, practitioners eliminate even their water and liquid consumption. However, they are free to eat normally within the dietary restrictions of Islam during the meal hours at night and throughout the rest of the year.

- Due to the risk of severe digestive distress, potentially life-threatening dehydration and metabolic issues associated with increased calorie consumption during the evening hours just before bed, this form of fasting is not recommended for those interested in using it as a means of improving their overall strength and wellness.

Christians are not required to fast for their religion but have used fasting for centuries as a means of getting closer to God. The practice is believed to prove an individual's true dedication, serve as a proper act of penance, and strengthen their personal commitment through sacrifice and self-control. Though forty days is the standard amount of time for experienced fasters, some Christians fast only on the holy day of Sunday while others fast throughout the Catholic celebration of Lent.

Buddhism is another belief system famous for fasting as a form of devotion and discipline. It promotes a consistent style of Intermittent Fasting where people only eat in the early hours of the morning, then start fasting at noon and continue to do so until the early hours of the next morning. The purpose of this is to practice self-discipline. When practiced as a lifestyle and not just as a temporary health plan, this has many physical and mental health benefits.

- Still, it is another form of Intermittent Fasting that is not recommended by medical professionals and other health experts to be used as a means of weight loss. It can cause an initial shock to your system that can increase fluid retention and fat storage in the body cells, and thus can be challenging to adjust to.

Credit for the first use of fasting as a means of health improvement can be given to Hippocrates of Kos, a physician of ancient Greece, who is known as the father of modern medicine. He was the inspiration for the Hippocratic Oath. This oath is a pledge that new doctors take before they start their career – promising to uphold high ethical standards and never cause any harm to another human being.

One of Hippocrates' most commonly assigned treatments was to sip apple cider vinegar in place of regular food consumption for a few days to a week, depending on the severity of the original illness or discomfort. The reason behind this was it was assumed the cause of the original sickness was something foul or tainted the patient had consumed, which subsequently affected the digestive tract and then spread throughout the body.

By not eating until the symptoms cleared, the patient's body was given the opportunity to heal without the risk of consuming anything else toxic or fueling the sickness with calories and carbohydrates. The apple cider vinegar fought off starvation and kept the body functioning during the fasting period.

Intermittent Fasting Tip: Apple Cider Vinegar

Apple cider vinegar is recommended even today for its detoxifying effects and several other positive health benefits.

- When consumed regularly, apple cider vinegar helps to **balance pH levels** in the body. This enhances digestion, lowers blood sugar levels, and helps to boost energy.
- Apple cider vinegar has also been praised for its effectiveness in **fighting cardiovascular diseases** and improving overall heart health.
- Since it is **full of natural antioxidants**, apple cider vinegar also helps to strengthen the body's immune system.
- **For Women:** Apple cider vinegar also strengthens the bones and joints. This is the reason it is recommended for women since females tend to have more significant issues with skeletal degeneration over time than males do.
- Many doctors and dieticians recommend female patients consume one or two tablespoons of apple cider vinegar per day, diluted in water or undiluted depending on personal preference. Whether or not a

woman decides to start fasting or go with a particular diet program, regular consumption of apple cider vinegar to improve bone health is still a good habit to pick up.

Another theory as to why the apple cider vinegar diet and fasting plan was (and still is) so effective is that avoiding food when feeling under the weather is a natural instinctive response. People tend to avoid heavy meals and gravitate towards hot tea and broth-based soups when they are not feeling well. Thus pairing lighter and liquid-based diets with fasting works well in such cases.

What Happens to the Food You Eat?

The human body has two main settings/mechanisms that determine how smoothly our internal systems run. These mechanisms provide energy to the body throughout the day and provide extra fuel from stored fat cells to injured areas of the body to speed up the healing process.

#1 Store Fat for Later Use: When people consume carbohydrates, sugars, and excess protein, the body digests it and uses it for the energy and nutrition it needs at the present moment. Then it transfers the remainder to the liver to get converted into glycogen that can be stored in fat deposits around the body in case of emergency. This is the process most active in the human body during feeding or feasting windows when food is being consumed regularly. When humans eat, the insulin production levels of the body increase, thanks to the consumed sugars being digested and deposited in the liver as fat cells. When the liver itself can't hold any more fat, but the human continues to eat, all new fat created from ingested food travels to other storage areas such as the core and thighs.

#2 **Burn Stored Fat for Extra Fuel:** This process is the one that is most active in times of fasting. Instead of relying on glucose delivered from food sources, the body can call upon stored fat cells to convert into emergency energy for the internal organs or body processes. This is the body's natural survival defense against starvation and can happen in times of distress, such as being lost or at the mercy of harsh weather. It is also a process that can be initiated and controlled without risk of fatality or illness with the help of Intermittent Fasting. It is monitored and upheld by a person's fluctuating glucose levels. When this begins, the body switches from running on empty sugar cells to burning excess fat so it can maintain energy, until the individual eats again.

Intermittent Fasting or IF works by creating (and sticking to) a fasting schedule designed to control the body when it slips in and out of these two processes to minimize fat storage and maximize fat burning.

Intermittent Fasting Tip: Fasting Is Habit & Determination, Not A Miracle Cure

Intermittent Fasting works as a valuable weight loss and health improvement tool only when it is done properly. This means taking the time to make a plan (something the guide will cover in the next chapter) and accepting that IF is not something that is recommended for use in short bursts.

There are those who will argue that the term "intermittent" encourages short-term use, however, in the case of Intermittent Fasting, this term is referring to the shorter fasting windows spread throughout each week of fasting, and not how long an individual is deciding to fast.

For example, someone takes part in one or two weeks of fasting to reach a particular weight loss goal and then abandons their fasting schedule. Typically, what happens is that when the individual returns to their pre-fasting lifestyle, the weight comes back because the body starts to refill those burned off fat stores, it lost during the fasting windows.

Intermittent Fasting is most effective and beneficial when it is undertaken as a lifestyle change. This is particularly true for those with pre-existing health conditions that are related to or can be affected by how the body changes with periods of fluctuating food consumption and deprivation.

Not only does adapting IF into one's daily lifestyle build it as a habit, but it also gives the body some sense of schedule and consistency. Remaining firm in a personalized Intermittent Fasting schedule also gives fasters an excellent opportunity to ensure they enjoy all the health benefits fasting can provide.

The Science of Intermittent Fasting: How Does It Work?

When you eat a meal, your body works a couple of hours to process the food, burning what you can from what you just consumed. Because you have all this amount of food available, it is easy for your body to use it to generate energy, instead of using stored fat. This is especially true when you consume carbohydrates/sugars since our bodies prefer to burn sugar as energy before any other source.

But, during the "fasting state," your body does not have stored food to use as energy, so instead of the glucose in the bloodstream or the glycogen stored in the muscles, you are more likely to use the stored fat in your body.

Objective achieved = Fat burning.

The same process happens if you do exercise during "fasting." Without a supply of glucose and glycogen to be used as energy (which has already been depleted during fasting, and which has not yet been replenished with food before training), the body is forced to adapt and use the only source of energy available: the fat stored in your cells.

Your body is sensitive to insulin after a period of fasting. Since Glycogen (a starch saved in the muscles and liver that your body can burn as fuel when needed) is exhausted during fasting and is depleted even more during training, it further increases sensitivity to insulin. This means that when you eat immediately after your workout, it will be stored more efficiently: especially in the form of glycogen in the muscles, and with minimal amounts stored as fat.

Not only that, during Intermittent Fasting, the secretion of growth hormone also increases. And the combined effect of this increased growth hormone secretion and decrease in insulin production (along with an increase in insulin sensitivity) teaches your body to efficiently utilize the food you eat, thereby leading to weight loss and muscle development.

Why Should You Practice Intermittent Fasting?

Because Intermittent Fasting works. Though we know that not all calories are the same, still caloric restriction plays a vital role in weight loss. When you fast, either for 16 hours a day or 24 hours from time to time, you reduce your calorie intake, which gives your body the possibility to lose weight.

Intermittent Fasting also simplifies your day. It requires less time (and possibly less money). Instead of buying or preparing three or six meals a day, you will only have to make two meals. Instead of leaving what you are doing six times a day just to eat, you simply have to stop to eat twice. Instead of having to wash the dishes six times, you just have to do it twice. Instead of having to shop for six meals a day, you only have to buy for two.

Apart from that, as previously explained, IF also promotes insulin sensitivity and increases the secretion of growth hormone. This helps you to lose weight and increase muscle. In the following chapters, we will discuss the benefits of Intermittent Fasting in further details.

What are the Disadvantages of Intermittent Fasting?

The biggest problem and the biggest concern that most people have is that Intermittent Fasting causes low energy, low concentration, and a strong desire to eat during the fasting period. People worry that throughout the morning, they will be miserable because they have not eaten any food, and this will adversely affect their work and effectiveness in whatever task they do.

But you must realize that these negative thoughts arise due to overthinking. Though the initial transition from EATING ALL the TIME, and moving to Intermittent Fasting can be a bit complicated for your system, however, once you have made that transition to eating only a few times a day, your body will quickly adapt and learn to function that way.

Once you train your body to not wait for food all day every day (or first thing in the morning), these side consequences will become a minor problem, thanks to a substance that our body produces called ghrelin. So if you take in food every three hours, you will start feeling hungry every three hours, as your body will learn and get used to food every three hours.

Again, think of it in terms of a caveman. The only reason they could survive during periods of scarcity was fasting. Our body can survive 84 hours of fasting before our glucose levels are negatively affected. In IF, we are talking about only small fasts that range from 16 to 24 hours. So, don't worry! With a little bit of will power, you will also be able to practice Intermittent Fasting, and it will not harm you in the least.

Is Intermittent Fasting Suitable for All Women?

No, IF is not suitable for all women. But, it does not mean you should be scared now and not try IF. For 99% of women, it works perfectly well. It just means that you have to be a little more careful.

If you are experiencing any of the following scenarios, then stay away from Intermittent Fasting:

- Your period is suspended
- You have sleep problems
- You are in a state of anxiety
- Your recovery after training worsens
- Hair fall increases
- Your body feels colder than normal
- Your mood keeps getting worse
- Your skin feels irritated
- You have less desire for sex

Also, Intermittent Fasting should not be practiced by pregnant women. The explanation is simple. As soon as the fetus is in the mother's womb, it always secures its nutrients no matter what consequences this may have for the mother. The fetus is fighting for its survival. For this reason, pregnancy at the wrong time - e.g., during a hunger (= fasting) period can end badly for the mother.

The best tip to successfully carry out Intermittent Fasting is to listen to your body. In the subsequent chapters, we will discuss about IF routines, the benefits, mindset, types of diets, and much more.

Once you start Intermittent Fasting, you'll soon realize if it is right for you, and that does not mean you should give up after 1-2 days just because you're hungry during fasting, which is normal as long as your body is not used to it.

IF is an excellent strategy to lose weight quickly and painlessly and to live longer at the same time. But the fact is it varies from person to person. For most, it works perfectly well and for some, not at all. You just have to try it yourself.

Chapter 2

Intermittent Fasting for Women

Now that I have covered the basics of Intermittent Fasting as a health enhancement option, let us dive into the specifics of IF and discuss how it relates to females and their personal health. Women who have been working out or dieting throughout the course of their lives know not every program that works for males gives similar outcomes for females, despite following the same steps, routine or dietary regimen.

In this chapter, we will take a look at some of the differences in Intermittent Fasting between male and female participants, introduce the first two steps of our simple 6-step process to mastering IF, and provide some helpful tips and tricks to get started on your own IF journey!

Intermittent Fasting & The Female Form

There are a number of factors, from the biological to the hormonal, that can affect the success of any dieting, nutrition, or fitness program for women. Some of the harmful effects and risks that women see more than men do when starting a new Intermittent Fasting routine include:

- **Hormonal imbalance:** Hormonal imbalances in females can evolve into a wide variety of more pressing concerns related to biology and genetics. Some of these concerns include irregular menstruation (length of period or strength of flow), changes in skin tone and sudden, difficult to clear blemishes.

- **Excessive fatigue:** Fatigue and muscle weakness are two common side effects associated with reduced calorie intake, but for women, these adverse reactions get magnified as the female body relies more on glucose and fat storage to function. While over time the negative effects decrease or even disappear, the initial transition and adaptation to a fasting schedule (also depending on how intense the fasting plan is) is typically more difficult for women in the first few weeks.
- **Emotional instability:** Also, often related to fluctuating hormones, mood swings are a common problem reported by women following an Intermittent Fasting plan, especially in the first two weeks to one month.

But, it's not all health concerns and difficulties! There are a lot of ways by which females can benefit from adding IF to their daily dietary schedule and develop it as a part of their lifestyle to enhance their overall health.

How Does Intermittent Fasting Benefit Women?

Women who have high cholesterol levels, existing heart conditions or are at a considerable risk of heart diseases have praised Intermittent Fasting since it has improved their current health conditions (along with the guidance of a personal physician or medical professional). But, these are just a few of the many health benefits that have been revealed by women who have adopted IF in their daily lifestyle.

Other widely reported positive health effects include:

Increased insulin sensitivity.

- **Reduced food cravings** by maintaining normal levels of the "hunger hormone," Ghrelin.
- **Boosting autophagy**, the natural cleansing mechanism by which the body cells clear out and recycle old, unwanted cellular components to restore proper functioning of all cellular processes.
- **Effective treatment of Type 2 Diabetes** and other blood sugar-related conditions. This is possible due to the increased insulin production the body experiences as a result of Intermittent Fasting.

Suppressed inflammations.

- **Reduced risk of obesity** owing to improvements in body composition and metabolic efficiency by burning visceral fat.
- Tremendous **improvements in the symptoms of auto-immune diseases** such as Crohn's disease, Systemic Lupus Erythematosus (SLE), rheumatoid arthritis, and colitis.
- **Lowered blood pressure** and greater control over blood pressure-related conditions.

Improved functioning of the pancreas.

- **Increased production of ketone bodies,** thereby enhancing cognitive function and protecting against neurological diseases like dementia, Parkinson's disease, and Alzheimer's disease.
- **Reduced risk of cancer.** Cancer cells are more receptive to insulin than normal cells. Since Intermittent Fasting promotes insulin sensitivity, it starves the cancer cells and leaves them vulnerable to destruction.
- **Higher production of HGH or fitness hormone.** This hormone is crucial in increasing longevity and maintaining optimum health by

boosting metabolism, burning fat pockets, and promoting muscle development.

In addition to all the benefits mentioned above, Intermittent Fasting also helps women who are in their menopause stages, lose the extra weight gained due to hormonal fluctuations. Not only that, practicing IF also makes you emotionally stable and empowers you to control your emotional impulses throughout the day.

Though its full effects are still being studied on human participants, in the last decade, tests featuring the impact of IF on female rats, in their menopausal stage, have shown encouraging results. Thus Intermittent Fasting is being widely recommended for women who struggle to control their menopause symptoms.

While the health benefits of IF are promising, specifically for women, it is essential to remember that a number of variables affect the effectiveness of fasting schedules and everyone's experience with fasting will be different depending on their personal health, biological makeup, lifestyle, and diet.

How Is Intermittent Fasting Riskier for Women?

Female participants in studies across the globe, and those communicating their personal results on social media or within fitness communities report many of the same negative effects felt by men throughout the course of adjusting to a new Intermittent Fasting plan. Some of these side effects include:

- Initial hunger pangs and dehydration
- Difficulty in concentrating or gaining focus throughout the day
- Headaches, muscle weakness, initial loss in muscle tone

Apart from these, women who have a history of irregular menstrual cycles have reported experiencing some symptoms of infertility after continuing Intermittent Fasting for a considerable span of time. This tendency is more common among females who see a dramatic loss in body fat, especially in the first few weeks (or during the adjustment period) of their IF schedule.

- However, such changes are never permanent, so there is nothing to be concerned about. Typically periods return to normal, and fertility increases in the weeks after stopping the Intermittent Fasting plan.

- Most wellness experts and medical professionals also recommend that women who are pregnant or are hoping to become pregnant in the near future avoid starting or cease their IF plan in order to ensure they do not minimize their chances of conceiving and are in peak condition for childbearing.

It is important to point out that even though IF is still being studied around the world for its potential long-term advantages and risks on nearly anyone (irrespective of age, gender, race, health histories), health and wellness experts all over the medical community have written and spoken about its safety, benefits and future possibilities for men and women alike. It all comes down to being prepared, having all the right information, and making a strategy that you can confidently stick to in the long run.

Step One: Making A Plan That Will Get Results

When starting your IF routine, it is crucial to remember that the best results come from creating a long-term plan. Intermittent Fasting is not designed to be used as an overnight or short-term weight loss method. In fact, people who do that end up developing eating disorders.

There is a difference between fasting and starving. There is a difference between intentionally avoiding food in search of some kind of miraculous cure and Intermittent Fasting as a lifestyle change.

Also, another thing that is important to remember is to consult a medical professional before undertaking any form of major change in terms of your personal health.

Asking the Right Questions

When creating your IF schedule, there are a number of questions that you must ask yourself, such as:

- What are my short-term health goals (three to six months) and long-term health goals (one year and beyond)?
- This could be to lose a certain number of pounds or inches with the help of Intermittent Fasting. It could also be less specific fitness-wise such as becoming fit enough to tackle a certain trail in your area or maybe to be able to walk a marathon.
- Have I chosen the right IF method for meeting my personal needs and goals?

- Is fasting the best option for me?
- Have I spoken to my personal physician or another medical professional to ensure a safe transition into and consistency with Intermittent Fasting in the long-term?
- Is the plan I've laid out realistic with respect to my current health status and existing conditions, as well as for reaching my personal health goals?
- Have I weighed the benefits versus the risks of starting an IF plan and determined what I can do to make the transition as easy as possible before starting?

As soon as these questions are fully answered, each person has what they need to take their first steps toward success with an Intermittent Fasting lifestyle.

Gather All the Information You Can

Creating a plan is the perfect way for first-time fasters and anyone curious about trying IF to get a good idea of how their body will react to longer fasting windows without worrying about the negative side effects like excessive fatigue that can come with an abrupt switch to the program.

This is particularly true for those who have decided not to ease themselves in by cutting back on one meal or a couple of hundred calories at a time in the weeks preceding their first official fasting window.

Before planning your first major fasting window or initiating an Intermittent Fasting plan, find out all the information you can on fasting, on fitness, and on diets that work with fasting schedules to maximize health benefits.

To take it a step further, make a list of questions you have concerning IF, its planning and preparation stages and consult a local gym or any healthcare professional to find out the answers. In case some questions remain unanswered, try searching for the solutions on the internet, but always remember to gather information from reliable websites only.

The more information you have at your disposal, the easier it will be for you to create a routine that is easier to stick to and delivers the most health benefits with the least side effects.

Determine Your Motivation & Set Realistic Goals

Before beginning any kind of diet or fitness routine, it is important to understand why you want to undertake the change, and all that comes with it. Just because a new health trend is taking the world by storm, it does not mean that it is the best option for everyone or that it will work for everyone.

Any form of diet or fitness routine requires adaptability, focus, determination, and sacrifice. This is one reason why it is a good idea to determine, if not write out, your motivations for wanting to start an Intermittent Fasting routine.

Not only will this help with setting goals, but it will also provide an excellent means of support and motivation on days when temptation comes calling, or there's been a trip up in your plans, thereby ultimately interrupting your fasting schedule.

Once you know why you want to try Intermittent Fasting, it's time for you to set your health goals and expectations for the routine you're planning to start. Where do you want to be in one month, three months, six months, and a year?

In the beginning, you might be unsure about how quickly your body will adapt to IF along with any other programs you may be trying with it (such as a specific diet or exercise routine). But if you set goals, it will give you a starting point that you can come back to any time you need to make adjustments to your schedule.

Getting Your Body Accustomed To Fasting

The best way to start Intermittent Fasting (particularly for those who have never attempted it or attempted it without success before) is to ease your body into it by restricting daily calorie consumption and skipping a meal every day for a week. This makes it less of a shock to the system and the body can take its time adjusting to switching between fat storing and fat burning processes smoothly, without upsetting the digestive system.

Once you've seen how your body reacts to skipping a meal and reducing calorie intake, then you can go ahead and lessen another hundred calories a day or eat lighter meals in place of the ones you aren't skipping.

In addition to getting your body used to the IF schedule, minimizing calorie intake before beginning a long-term fasting routine will also allow you to prepare yourself mentally. You'll be able to fully embrace and appreciate the purpose of Intermittent Fasting, and will feel more in control of the new habits and challenges that come with starting a fasting health program.

Intermittent Fasting Tip: The Best First Step Is the Baby Step

This is true for any kind of major lifestyle, diet, or fitness change. Sudden changes can send the body into episodes of mild shock that can either clear up with time and determination or escalate into more significant health concerns.

Those who look at IF as a quick fix to a particular concern or condition will typically see less progress and benefits than those who accept it as a change in lifestyle for the betterment of their overall health and wellness.

Easing oneself into a personalized Intermittent Fasting plan comes with a number of benefits, including:

- An easier time tweaking, fine-tuning, and adjusting your IF schedule to combat side effects or maximize health benefits.
- More time to monitor how the body is reacting to fasting as a regular part of life so that adjustments can be made to ease discomfort or clear potential negative effects.
- Being mentally prepared for the physical and social changes your life will

undergo as a result of following a regular fasting routine.

It is easy to get excited at the start of any new health journey, but with Intermittent Fasting, the more time you invest in understanding the feelings and changes the body is trying to communicate, the more likely will you see long-term success with your personalized (and continuously developing) fasting plan.

Step Two: Choosing A Realistic Intermittent Fasting Plan

Choosing a schedule that you can stick to for a long duration is fundamental in finding success in life.

One of the reasons people fall in love with Intermittent Fasting is how adaptable it is to almost any kind of daily schedule. With a variety of popular methods that range in time frames, calorie intake, or the number of days they last, anyone can find an IF routine that works for them.

However, it is essential to remember that the vital part of laying out a personalized, yet realistic IF plan is to find a fasting routine that will work with your current daily schedule on a more prolonged basis, and not just for one to two weeks.

Keeping that in mind, in chapter 5, I'll discuss eight popular ways of Intermittent Fasting that can help you to achieve a body that you feel more confident about.

All of them can be effective, but which one will suit you the best will depend on your lifestyle and how committed you are to becoming a healthier version of yourself.

But, before that, we'll talk about the findings of some scientific studies that have been carried out in this domain.

Also, we'll discuss about the process that is responsible for the miraculous effects of Intermittent Fasting, "autophagy". Therefore, keep reading!

Chapter 3

Intermittent Fasting: Benefits, Side Effects & Precautions

Without self-control, you cannot be confident. If you happen to sabotage yourself continually, rather than becoming confident, you'll experience an internal conflict. However, when you act in ways intended, such as completing a fast, your confidence level will increase, and you'll start developing greater trust in your capabilities. This will prompt you to take bigger risks and set bigger goals and challenges in the future.

A study carried out on mice in the year 2003 confirmed that fasting helps to develop resistance to stress and lead a longer life. Also, the best available research, which was published in 2016, suggests that a controlled act of abstinence from food slows down aging.

Although withdrawal or abstinence from food is a physical challenge, the rewards that come with it also include spiritual growth and psychological well-being. Fasting is about challenging yourself. It helps you to grow as an individual and reach a state of self-actualization. It also allows you to be more at peace with yourself and your environment. Religion-wise, fasting brings you closer to God, as it opens doors to prayer and meditation.

Research has shown that fasting can help to reset your sleep cycle and enhance the quality of your sleep. Fasting also improves your psychological health. It reduces the risk of stroke and post-stroke brain damage.

Aging Process

The restriction of calorie intake (calorie restriction, CR) is one of the most reliable methods to significantly increase the lifespan of various organisms from yeast, worms to nonhuman primates.

CR generally means a 10-30% reduction in daily calorie intake. It is associated with improved insulin sensitivity, lowering of heart rate and blood pressure (which benefits cardiovascular health), reduced free radical damage to cellular components (proteins, DNA), reduced incidence of spontaneous and induced tumors, and better resistance to neurodegenerative diseases.

Intermittent Fasting is an alternative to calorie restriction, with a similar effect on the aging process and lifespan. When fasting was introduced at a young age in rats, it resulted in an extension of their average lifespan by 2.8-6.7 months.

A similar thing also happens to humans. When you fast, due to the calorie withdrawal, your body goes under stress and releases a whole lot of chemicals that not only protect you from the side effects that come with abstaining from food but also help to fight depression and anxiety. Scientists believe it is due to these chemicals that our bodies develop increased stress resistance, which ultimately slows down aging and extends our longevity.

Lowered Cardiovascular Risk

In one study, Intermittent Fasting in non-obese participants showed an increase in good HDL cholesterol in women and a reduction in triglyceride levels in men. This effect occurred over a span of 22 days, during which the participants fasted every two days. The change was caused due to the degradation of body fat by 4%.

In the case of obese people, the values improved more clearly by an average weight loss of 5.6 kg after eight weeks of Intermittent Fasting.

Total cholesterol levels dropped by 21%, LDL cholesterol by 25% and triglycerides by 32%, while HDL cholesterol remained unchanged.

The systolic blood pressure dropped from 124 to 116 mmHg.

Beyond reducing body weight, stress resistance induced by Intermittent Fasting also has a cardioprotective effect. Studies in mice show that in a heart attack, the affected heart area is half times smaller in alternately fasting mice than in normally fed animals. Also, in cardiac infarction, four times fewer cardiomyocytes (heart muscle cells) died, when the animals were fed intermittently.

Intermittent Fasting For Cancer Prevention

Intermittent Fasting reduces the development and progression of malignant tumors. Rats on IF, transplanted with a cancer cell line, survived longer than their free-fed counterparts. After ten days, 50% of the IF animals were still alive compared to the other 12.5% in the control group.

IF, performed in middle-aged rats, saw the reduced incidence of lymphoma as well. In a 4-month observation period, 30% of the control mice became ill while none of the animals on the IF routine became cancerous. Intermittent Fasting also reduced the development of pre-neoplastic (precursor to cancer) liver injury and liver nodules caused by carcinogenic substances.

The researchers also found a better antioxidant activity among the fasting rats, which resulted in less development of harmful free radicals within the mitochondria (cell power plants). This antitumor effect did not result from the calorie reduction since both groups consumed the same amount of calories.

Brain Power and Aging

Intermittent Fasting boosts neuronal functionality, which is a process that decreases with age.

With advancing age, the dendritic spines, which are small membranous protrusions from a neuron's (nerve cell's) dendrite, decrease. These spines play a vital role in the information transfer between the nerve cells. However, with growing age, as the number of these spines reduce, the efficiency of neural processes also become adversely affected.

Intermittent Fasting prevents the reduction of the density of these spines. In rats, that lived on a normal diet, the number of spines decreased by 38% after 24 months of observation. But, the rats that were under an IF routine showed little difference to a young, 6-month-old rat even after 24 months. In fact, these rats showed an improvement in their learning abilities.

Calorie reduction, caused due to Intermittent Fasting increases neurogenesis (formation of new brain cells), protects the neurons from dying and stimulates the production of BDNF (Brain-Derived Neurotrophic Factor), a protein associated with increased neurogenesis, Therefore, IF slows down the neuron degenerative processes, and thus aging.

The effect on neurogenesis also appears to promote healing and functional recovery of spinal cord injuries in animals, whether Intermittent Fasting is introduced before or shortly after the injury.

Calorie Independent Effect

IF can have a positive effect on health and life expectancy, as we have discussed so far. Some Intermittent Fasting researchers and advocates claim that because fasting is a kind of stress for the body, it could stimulate the expression of genes that perform protective tasks and theoretically bring health benefits.

Some nutritionists argue that our ancestors did not consistently have food supplies, but were instead exposed to hunger periods and periods of increased caloric intake and that their genes were shaped and adapted accordingly. Thus, an alternate availability of food would be "natural."

IF partially dissociates the positive effects of calorie reduction from the actual total intake of calories. In mice, Intermittent Fasting results in improved glucose control, lower insulin levels, and higher resistance to neuronal damage regardless of weight loss or calorie intake.

Even without a reduction in calories, Intermittent Fasting increases the concentration of the hormone Adiponectin. Adiponectin is a protein hormone that promotes fat burning, possesses anti-inflammatory and anti-diabetic properties, and has a positive influence on cardiovascular health.

Side Effects of Intermittent Fasting

Everyone fasts for various reasons – to lose weight, for a religious purpose, for healthy living and the list goes on. A fast could either be mild or strict (ranging from liquid only such as juice, tea, coffee and the likes to no food, no fluid). Although fasting comes with a lot of benefits, it also has its associated downsides, that vary from one individual to another.

- **Poor weight management:** Many people tend to crave for and consume more calories after a long period of fast, which inevitably counteracts all the progress made by fasting.
- **Short-term downsides:** Intermittent Fasting can have several short-lived adverse effects such as dizziness, headaches, outbursts, weakness, low blood pressure, gouts, and gall stones.

- **Long-Term downsides:** Continuous prolonged fasting could weaken the immune system and affect vital organs such as the kidneys and the liver. When an individual abstains from food over a long period, the person becomes malnourished. This could lead to an untimely death after the entire energy store of the body gets exhausted.

Precautions to Take

Intermittent Fasting has a lot of advantages. However, it is not meant for everyone. To better understand the theory of fasting, let us compare it to a tool, such as an arrow, which can either be used properly or misused.

A hunter could have different sizes and tips of arrows in his quiver. When he finds an antelope, he would use a sharp wooden arrow, but when faced by a lion or bear, he would go for something stronger: probably an arrow with metallic tips. The point is, do not use the wrong method for the right purpose.

Who Should Avoid Intermittent Fasting?

- **Pregnant and breastfeeding mothers** should stay away from IF. Both the mother and the infant need to be fed well to stay nourished and healthy. Whether you have a child who you're breastfeeding or one who is still in your uterus, you need all the calories you can get.

- **Youngsters under the age of 18** are still growing and need all the vital nutrients and minerals for their growth and development. Hence they must refrain from practicing IF.
- Intermittent Fasting is also not meant for people who are **underweight or malnourished.** If you find it difficult to tell whether you are malnourished or not, you can ask your physician or a trusted friend. Those having an eating disorder such as bulimia are also included in this category.
- Another group of individuals who might want to give IF a miss is those with occasional **gastroesophageal reflux disease (GERD)**. There are solid pieces of evidence to prove that GERD could be aggravated by fasting. This possible worsening is because during fasting, the stomach remains devoid of food and there is nothing which the gastric juices can digest.

Who Needs To Be Cautious?

- **Individuals who have Type-2 Diabetes** need to consult your physician before beginning Intermittent Fasting.
- **Individuals on medications** need to be careful during IF as the fasting periods could overlap with those drugs that require one to eat before having them.
- In addition, those on **cancer therapy** and other medical treatment must be cautious and should have an in-depth discussion with their physician before starting Intermittent Fasting.

Chapter 4

Autophagy Revolution

Do you suffer from recurrent body pains? Are you easily prone to illness? Do you find it challenging to shed weight? Then, all you need to do is to acquire more knowledge about autophagy and the fasting processed involved.

Autophagy ranks high among the most popular methods of weight management and healthy living for a reason. Most people who have tried it, swear by the benefits they have derived and the ways it has improved their lives. But then, what is autophagy?

- Derived from the combination of two words, 'auto' which means self and 'phagein' which means to engulf, autophagy is defined as the process of engulfment of harmful microbes, damaged cell organelles (specialized subunits found within a cell) and other unwanted cellular components, to either eliminate them or recycle them. It is a biological process by which new cells can regenerate, and your body can be detoxified.

If such cells and pathogens are not removed from your body in a timely manner, it may reduce your life span, by causing neurodegenerative, inflammatory, cardiovascular, and other types of diseases.

The Origin of Autophagy

Christian de Duve, a Belgian scientist, first coined the term "autophagy" while studying lysosomes and the role of glucagon (a peptide hormone responsible for raising the blood sugar level) in cell degradation.

Between 1970 and 1980, researchers began taking a closer look at the process of cellular autophagy. At that time, little information was available about the importance of this process.

After many years of hard work, a significant milestone was achieved in 1983, when Yoshinori Ohsumi, discovered the genes responsible for the regulation of autophagy in yeast. From his discovery, he found that autophagy was absent in yeast cells lacking those genes, and such cells were unable to repair themselves. In 2016, he was awarded a Nobel Prize for this great discovery.

The interesting thing about Ohsumi's discovery is how cells typically respond to increased stress, nutrient deficiency, deprivation of energy, and cellular injuries by increasing the rate of cellular autophagy (stress response mode). But when the stress is eliminated, the process of autophagy goes back to the regular rate (maintenance mode).

To fully understand autophagy, more research works are now aimed at studying the relationship between aging and autophagy, and the effect of stress on this process.

According to evidence, the process that enhances autophagy can also help to extend the lifespan of individuals. It is believed that cell aging occurs when unwanted cellular components start accumulating and are not properly removed.

Since autophagy helps to remove damaged cell materials, it might be able to slow down the process of aging. Hence scientists are looking for ways of extending the life expectancy of humans by inducing autophagy.

The Benefits of Autophagy

Over time, the metabolic activities in a healthy human body cause cellular damage. Sadly, the rate at which your cells are damaged increases as you age due to stress, poor diet, exposure to radiation, and other factors.

However, autophagy eliminates such damaged and old cells that are no longer active but are still present in the body. It also helps the cells to get rid of infection-causing pathogens. As a result, this leads to a number of health benefits:

- Autophagy can **extend the average lifespan** of humans.

Cells are the building blocks of life, and autophagy helps to remove the waste materials from these blocks. With the toxic substances gone, the metabolic efficiency of the cells improve, and they become healthy.

In addition to this, autophagy also helps the body to deal with stress.

- Psychiatric diseases like **depression and schizophrenia can be prevented** using autophagy.
- It also helps to **protect from neurodegenerative disorders** like Alzheimer's disease, Parkinson's disease, and dementia.
- It **strengthens the immune system** and protects you from infections by destroying harmful microbes, and removing toxins from inside the cells.
- Lastly, autophagy can **prevent the onset of cancer** and can even inhibit the growth of early-stage cancers.

The Process of Autophagy

There are three main methods by which autophagy occurs. They are:

- Macroautophagy
- Microautophagy
- Chaperone-mediated autophagy **(CMA)**

All the three forms involve transporting the cellular waste materials to the lysosome (a cell organelle that contains enzymes required for autophagy) to be broken down and recycled.

Macroautophagy: During this process, all waste materials within a cell are transported via a double membrane-bound vesicle (called an autophagosome) to the lysosome. The autophagosome then fuses with the lysosome and empties its contents, so that the waste materials can be processed.

Microautophagy: This is in sharp contrast with the process of macroautophagy. In this case, the cellular wastes to be digested are not transported via any vesicle, but rather, they are mopped up by the lysosome itself, by either developing cellular protrusions or invagination (inward folding of an area of the lysosomal membrane.)

Chaperone-mediated autophagy: During this process, the cell utilizes chaperone proteins (such as Hsc-70) which are found on the surface of the lysosomal membrane. These chaperones bind to the unwanted protein molecules within the cell, forming a chaperone/substrate complex. This complex molecule then attaches with the lysosome wall to allow the protein molecules to enter the lysosome for disintegration.

In each of these three procedures, both selective and non-selective degradation techniques are employed, depending on the organelle or molecule that needs to be recycled or broken down.

In the end, the cellular components to be degraded are collected within the lysosome and converted into smaller/micro molecules such as fatty acids, amino acids, glucose, and nucleotides.

These micro molecules are then reused by the cell to form larger molecules and new cell organelles. In this way, autophagy rejuvenates the body cells and makes you feel better, younger, and healthier.

Autophagy Vs. Apoptosis

Apoptosis is defined as the programmed death of a cell which occurs as part of the cell's normal activities.

Cell death occurs to ensure a balance between good and healthy cells and those that are senescent.

But one may wonder how apoptosis is related to autophagy. Researchers are particularly interested in the association between autophagy and apoptosis because they believe that such knowledge could aid the treatment of cancer and management of neurodegenerative diseases such as Alzheimer's disease due to the capacity of both the processes to regulate cell death. When such knowledge is available, autophagy could be used as a therapeutic tool to eliminate harmful cells while protecting the healthy ones.

How to Induce Autophagy?

Autophagy is a survival mechanism and occurs in virtually all the cells in our body. However, in response to specific situations such as hunger/fasting, exercise, energy deficiency, and cellular injuries, our body experiences an increase in the stress levels, and this increased stress activates autophagy.

Pieces of fossil evidence from the past show strong, healthy bones and teeth of humans at an early stage of our history. However, there are also evidences to prove that our ancestors were able to survive for days without food.

So, how is it possible that they managed to stay fit without surplus food supplies, yet today, we face so many health issues?

Some reasons responsible for this include:

- **Hard work:** The early men had to farm or hunt before they could eat, unlike today, when you can easily stroll to a grocery store to buy foodstuffs. Thus our ancestors lead an active life, that involved doing plenty of physical tasks and workout. And exercise is indispensable if you want to stay healthy.
- **Lack of food/Fasting:** Yes, you read that right. Due to the lack of food in the past, our ancestors had to opt for fasting. This resulted in energy deficiency, which ultimately triggered autophagy and helped our ancestors survive the harsh conditions that prevailed in those times.

Here is a simple comparison between the ancient food environment and the modern food environment:

- **Accessibility:** Today, there is more than enough food for everyone to eat. Also, it is affordable and easily accessible to all.
- **You can eat anytime you want:** Since food is readily available, if you are not cautious,

you might find yourself munching one thing or another for most of the day, thereby causing unhealthy weight gain.

- **People no longer have to work hard to eat:** Most of us drive down to the grocery or take a short stroll to the store with money in our pocket, and voila, we can purchase whatever we desire to eat. As a matter of fact, high-calorie food items are the cheapest items on the shelf. We no longer have to farm or hunt before eating.

In our modern society, an average individual can't go a day without having food. However, we do not engage in sufficient rigorous activities that could help expend energy to become energy deficient.

In simple terms, our input is not equivalent to our output (i.e., what we take in does not equate what goes out). This is strikingly different from the eating environment in which our ancestors lived, and if they were given similar opportunity today, they would fall over each other to have a fill.

Anything that enhances autophagy can have positive effects on our body. Thus, in this day and age, the most important thing we need to focus on is finding ways to activate the process of autophagy.

Four ways of inducing autophagy while carrying out your normal daily activities are:

Intermittent Fasting

In our hectic lifestyles, it is sometimes a little relieving to know that you can still control your eating habits and your lifestyle. One of the best triggers of autophagy is something we have been discussing since the beginning of this book, i.e., Intermittent Fasting. It has been reported that IF can promote neuronal autophagy.

Since IF is a form of time-restricted fasting in which an individual abstains from food for a specified period, it closely resembles the fasting pattern of our ancestors.

Studies have shown that performing Intermittent Fasting for 1-2 days (24-48 hours) usually produces the best results. Another option is to have your usual meal at regular intervals, and then go on a 2-3 days fast. However, this is an impossible task for most people.

Still, most participants can fast for half a day (12 hours) or more without too much trouble, and this can be done by eating once or twice daily. For instance, if you had your last meal by 7 pm today, the next meal should be around 7 am tomorrow. That way, you would have fasted for 12 hours. You could then have the next meal by 7 pm.

Another type of IF routine that is popular among beginners is Alternate Day fasting. When it comes to alternate fasting, you can cut down on your calorie intake during the fasting periods by eating only 1-2 meals ($\leq$ 500 calories), and then on regular days, you can have your fill of calories.

Apart from these two, there are other types of Intermittent Fasting routines as well, which we will discuss, in details, in the upcoming chapters.

Ketogenic Diets

Ketogenic diets (KD) comprise of food substances that are very rich in fat but low in carbohydrates. This triggers the body to undergo the process of gluconeogenesis (a process in which the body derives energy from non-carbohydrate sources such as fat).

These diets produce an effect similar to fasting and can thus cause an increase in autophagy. Ketogenic diets are primarily effective at activating autophagy in the brain.

Some food suggestions for KD include eggs, avocado, fermented cheeses, seeds, nuts, butter, olive oil, fish, vegetables, vitamins, etc.

If you are struggling with Intermittent Fasting, then Ketogenic diets are an ideal alternative for you.

Exercise

Exercise is one of the best stressors that is capable of triggering autophagy. It stimulates the body to regenerate and produce new tissues by breaking down the old, worn out ones.

According to scientific reports, exercising can initiate autophagy in many organs at the same time, such as the liver, the muscles, the pancreas, and also in the adipocytes.

The amount of activity needed to stimulate autophagy is not yet clearly defined. However, it has been observed that 30 minutes of exercise is enough to trigger autophagy in the cardiac and skeletal muscles.

Sleep

Even though a vast majority of people replace their rest time with binge-watching television, doing more work, and hanging out with friends, our body works at its optimum when we acknowledge it's circadian rhythm or natural biological clock.

This clock controls the metabolic activities and the production of hormones. It also governs our sleeping cycles and regulates the process of autophagy.

Without adequate sleep, the circadian rhythm fails to function correctly. This slows down the process of autophagy and negatively affects our health.

Dry Fasting & Water Fasting

Apart from Intermittent Fasting, there are two other forms of fasting that many people undertake to activate autophagy. These are dry fasting and water fasting.

In this section, I'll discuss what these are and why I don't recommend them.

Dry Fasting

Dry fasting is a dangerous form of fasting in which an individual abstains from both solid food and fluids. Despite its harshness, this brutal fasting method is still quite popular.

Fasting is about staying away from calories, to enable your body to reset its metabolic activities. This, however, doesn't mean you should stay away from drinking water or specific teas, provided you don't add sugars, or you're selective about the natural sweeteners you add.

Since dry fasting prohibits you from drinking water during the fasting phase, I would advise you to stay away from it for your health's sake. Also, such form of brutal fasting can lead to death if other underlying factors such as exertions, heat, and the likes set in.

Water Fasting

Water Fasting is another popular fasting type. This form of fasting is known for its autophagous, weight loss, detox, and anti-aging benefits.

When doing a water fast, you can't by any means, eat any solid food. Also, you are not expected to drink anything else besides water. In water fasting, the average daily intake of water is about 2-3 liters.

This fast should last for a minimum of 24 hours, with the maximum being 72 hours. Water fasting beyond this period requires guidance and supervision by medical professionals because some health risks might come with it.

During water fasts, try not to get involved in any overwhelming physical work. Also, stay away from long-distance driving to avoid accidents.

The reasons to avoid water fasting are:

- **High tendency of losing the wrong type of weight:** This form of fasting only allows the intake of water but restricts one from taking in calories. Although an individual could lose up to 0.9 kg (2 pounds) with 24-72 hours of water fasting, sadly, such weight reduction can be due to a loss of carbohydrates, muscle mass, and even water.
- **Possible dehydration:** As funny as it may sound, water fasting could still cause dehydration because about 20-30 percent of our daily water intake comes from the food we eat. Thus, if we consume the same amount of water as we do on average days, we could experience some symptoms of dehydration such as light-headedness, dizziness, constipation, headaches, weakness, nausea, etc. To prevent such unwanted side effects, you will have to increase your water consumption.
- **Possibility of experiencing Orthostatic Hypotension:** This type of hypotension is usually common among those who fast. You might have experienced something similar when you get up suddenly, and then you feel dizzy or lightheaded. That feeling is caused by

a sudden drop in the blood pressure and can cause blackouts. If you think you are experiencing orthostatic hypotension, then it means your body is not compatible with water fasting.

- **Worsen certain medical conditions:** You should avoid water fasting if you have:
- Gout: Gout is caused by an accumulation of uric acid in the joints, and water fasting could increase its production.
- Chronic kidney disease: Those with chronic kidney condition should stay away from water fasting as it may worsen such condition.
- Heartburn: Heartburn may be induced by water fasting as the body keeps producing gastric acid, even though there is no solid food to digest.

Intermittent Fasting, Autophagy & Anti-Aging – The Intersection

Aging is a result of a decrease in the rate and amount of autophagy, leading to the accumulation of higher amounts of junks and cellular damage.

As organisms age, they experience a decrease in their autophagous capacities, which means that they cannot service and repair themselves as they used to any longer. Due to this, after some time (days or months or years), most of the cells become damaged or start malfunctioning, losing their ability to function at an optimal level. If this degradation gets to vital organs, death becomes inevitable.

Autophagy occurs in a cycle, fluctuating at different rates at different times of the day. An increased level of eating reduces autophagy, while fasting increases it.

Therefore, if the result of aging is a decreased rate of autophagy and an increase in damage accumulation, and the effect of fasting is an increased rate of autophagy, then fasting combats aging.

Anti-aging is the most significant benefit that comes with Intermittent Fasting. IF is, in fact, the most effective anti-aging strategy available.

If we keep eating all the time, we won't enter a fasting state, and will in principle, never speed up autophagy. Remember, eating constantly, or "grazing" is a pro-aging activity, so, don't eat all the time.

Chapter 5

8 Types of Intermittent Fasting Diets

People around the world are seeing massive success with Intermittent Fasting. The reason, undoubtedly, is the variety of IF methods that have been developed through study and experience to achieve any number of personal wellness goals.

But before we dive into the different forms of IF, here are some common facts regarding each of the types we will be discussing in this chapter:

- Every method of Intermittent Fasting brings some unique advantage to the table. However, there are a few shared benefits as well –
- Enhanced metabolic health
- Weight loss and better fat burning
- Improved insulin sensitivity and regulation of blood sugar
- Lower blood pressure
- Reduced inflammation
- Improved brain function and focus
- Increased lifespan and healthy aging
- Irrespective of the type of IF diet you choose, ensure that your meals have plenty of healthy whole foods, such as –
- Vegetables: Leafy greens, cauliflower, broccoli, tomatoes, cucumbers, etc.

- Fruits: Apples, bananas, pears, peaches, berries, oranges, etc.
- Whole grains: Quinoa, oats, barley, rice, buckwheat, etc.
- Proteins: Fish, meat, poultry, eggs, legumes, nuts, seeds, etc.
- Healthy fats: Olive oil, coconut oil, and avocados
- Drink plenty of water and keep yourself hydrated.
- Always drink unsweetened tea and coffee and calorie-free beverages to control your appetite.
- Avoid foods that contain artificial sweeteners and have fewer nutritional benefits such as –
- Processed foods: Packaged fruit juices, candy bars, fast food meals, margarine, potato chips, cookies, pastries, cakes, low-fat yogurt, and processed meat (pepperoni, sausage, bacon).
- Refined carbohydrates: White bread, pasta, white rice.
- Excess fats: Cheese, animal fats, cooking oils.

Now, with that done, let's take a closer look at some of the most popular, and effective types of IF, how they work, and who they work best for.

And yes, this is step two of the 6-step process to mastering IF, so do pay attention!

The 16/8 Method: A Popular Choice

16/8 or 16:8 Intermittent Fasting is also referred to as the Leangains Method. It involves restricting the consumption of food items and calorie-laden beverages to a window of eight hours per day and then abstaining from any form of food for the remaining 16 hours. This creates a feeding and fasting window each day, thus helping you to adopt IF into your daily schedule. It is recommended to perform high-intensity exercises (during the eating window) a few times a week to increase the benefits associated with this IF method.

You can practice the 16/8 technique once or twice per week to every day, depending on your preference.

- The simplest way to master this method is to skip breakfast and eat around noon or lunchtime each day. Doing this will automatically reduce your daily calorie intake by at least a quarter to maybe by a third.

Then from 12 pm, you'll get 8 hours to have your meals. The eating window would end just before bedtime for most people, which is excellent as most nutritionists and dieticians recommend not eating in the hours before bed and in the later hours of the evening.

- Another option is to eat between 9 am and 5 pm, and then begin fasting for the next 16 hours. This schedule will allow you to have a healthy breakfast around 9 am, a standard lunch around noon and a light early snack or dinner around 4 pm.

The above time table may not work for everyone. So it is crucial to point out that as long as

- the 16-hour and 8-hour windows are maintained,
- all excess binging is avoided, and
- the schedule is one that fits your lifestyle and
- supports your energy needs instead of causing hunger and fatigue during peak physical or mental activity, this method of Intermittent Fasting will yield positive results.

A similar, yet advanced version of this method is the **18:6 method,** in which you fast for 18 hours, and then have a 6-hour window to have your food.

For those who are concerned about the effects of consistent longer fasting windows on the female form, worry not! I'll introduce you to other options as well that you can choose from.

Advantages of 16/8 Method

- **Reduction in Inflammation:** A survey that analyzed more than 2000 women found that those who performed longer nighttime fasts (more than 13 hours and up to 16 hours), showed reduced levels of inflammation.
- **Lower Breast Cancer Risk:** Researchers have also found that fasting for more than 13 hours per night significantly reduces the risk of recurrence of breast cancer in women.
- **Retain Lean Body Mass:** Studies have also shown that 16:8 fast burns body fat without destroying lean mass. In addition to that, the diet also improves muscle endurance.

Disadvantages of 16/8 Method

- This diet is **not an instant fix for weight loss,** so if you're expecting immediate results, you might get disappointed.
- If you have a fast metabolism, you'll be **unable to resist the urge to eat** during the fasting cycle.
- **Avoid 16/8 diet if you have eating disorders** like binge eating and overeating since fasting encourages such restrictive behaviors.

An Ideal Option for Women of All Ages: The 5/2 Intermittent Fasting Plan

Also called the Fast Diet, the 5:2 Intermittent Fasting method was popularized by the British journalist Michael Mosley.

With this dieting method, participants need not completely eliminate their daily calorie intake during the fasting periods, but instead, they must reduce their calorie consumption to a small percentage (30-50%) of what they consume on their average feeding days. This makes the 5/2 an ideal starting point for those who want to ease themselves before trying a more extreme form of fasting.

During the Fast Diet, for five days of the week, you eat normally, without restricting your calorie intake. Then, on the remaining two days, you decrease your calorie consumption to nearly a quarter of your daily needs, that is, around 500 kcal per day for women (and 600 for men).

It's crucial to emphasize that eating "normally" does not in any way mean you can eat everything. If you eat junk food, you probably won't lose any weight, and may even end up gaining some pounds. So, during the eating window, follow a healthy diet and consume the same amount of food that you would eat if you hadn't been fasting at all.

For this method, you can choose whichever two days of the week you feel would be the most suitable as per your routine, as long as there is at least one non-fasting day in between them.

- One common way of executing the 5:2 IF diet is to fast on Mondays and Thursdays, with two to three small meals, and then eat normally for the rest of the week.

While practicing the Fast Diet, aim for high-intensity activities at least four days of the week. Just three session of high-intensity exercise done for seven minutes can reduce body fat, increase muscle strength, and improve endurance. On the other two days, do five minutes of push-ups and planks or 50 crunches to tone your muscles.

You can also train on a fast day so that your body is forced to burn up fat reserves rather than using energy from food. However, remember that you don't overdo and cause burn out – the point here is quality, not quantity.

Advantages of 5/2 Method

- The 5:2 Intermittent Fasting method is **designed for fasting newcomers** who have difficulty with more intensive fasting programs.
- This method is **recommended for women of all ages** as the eating, and non-eating windows not only encourage health benefits such as weight loss and fat burning but are also less likely to have an effect on menstrual cycles and hormone levels.

Disadvantages of 5/2 Method

- The Fast Diet **can cause nutritional deficiencies** if you don't stick to nutrient-dense foods on non-fasting days.
- It can also **encourage binge eating** and disrupt sleep patterns.

- **Athletes and busy people** may find that during the fasting days, they **do not get sufficient energy** to perform their daily tasks.
- The Fast Diet is **not meant for women who are pregnant or are nursing**. Also, if you've had eating disorders or are recovering from surgery and taking medications like warfarin, do not attempt this diet.

When your body adjusts to the 5/2 method, you will be ready to increase your fasting windows and switch to the next diets discussed here.

Now, I'll discuss two advanced versions of the 5/2 method:

- Crescendo Fasting
- Eat Stop Eat Method

Crescendo Fasting

Compared to males, female bodies are highly sensitive to the signals of starvation. As a result, long durations of fasting can cause hormonal imbalances, thereby leading to hunger pangs, fatigue, mood swings, and in some cases, even weight gain.

Crescendo Fasting is a highly effective form of Intermittent Fasting that is well-suited for women and is also less demanding on their bodies.

Like the 5/2 technique, in the Crescendo method, you will not be fasting every day. In fact, you will fast only on 2 or 3 non-consecutive days per week for 12 to 16 hours. Rest of the days, you can continue your regular eating schedule.

- So, let's say you start with two days per week. As per your convenience, you can choose any non-consecutive days, for example, Monday and Thursday or Tuesday and Friday.

Here, I'm assuming you decide to fast Monday and Thursday for 16 hours. This means you can apply the 16:8 rule, that is fasting for 16 hours, followed by eating within an 8-hour window.

So, for example, on Sunday you complete your dinner at 6 pm and then fast until 10 am the next morning, that is, Monday. For the remaining portion of Monday, and on Tuesday and Wednesday, you eat normally. But on Thursday, you wait 16 hours after dinner and then have your first meal.

- After two weeks, if you feel comfortable, you can add one more day to your fasting routine.

This means, you will now be performing this fast three times weekly on non-consecutive days, say for example, on Tuesday, Thursday, and Saturday.

For example, if you continue with the 16:8 method, you finish your dinner at 6 pm on Monday and don't eat again until 10 am on Tuesday. For the rest of Tuesday and on Wednesday, you eat according to your regular schedule. However, you wait 16 hours after dinner to have your first meal on Thursday. And then you repeat this again on Friday until 10 am on Saturday.

- If you feel confident, you may even switch to the 18:6 method of Intermittent Fasting on the fasting days. This means on the 2 to 3 days per week that you will be fasting, you will extend the duration of the fast to 18 hours and then have a 6-hour eating window.

Avoid heavy workouts on the fasting days, instead focus on light cardio or yoga. For the non-fasting days, you can do more intense exercise such as strength training and Burst/HIIT training.

Advantages of Crescendo Fasting

- Crescendo method **prepares you physically and mentally for other complicated** forms of IF such as Eat, Stop, Eat, Alternate Day Fasting, and the Warrior Method.

- Due to its **gentle approach on the female body,** this form of fasting preserves the hormonal balance, which plays a crucial role in every woman's life.
- Crescendo Fasting is also an **excellent method to burn those fat pockets** and slim down in a not-so-difficult manner.

Disadvantages of Crescendo Fasting

- If you **experience irregular menstrual cycles,** then you must stop practicing Crescendo fasting.
- Also, if you have **eating disorders,** then this kind of fasting is not for you.

Eat Stop Eat

Started by Brad Pilon, this method of fasting helps many people lose weight and boosts their body metabolism. The concept behind this method is based on the following: you can eat everything you want during the week, except for one or two days when you shouldn't eat anything for 24 hours. As long as this period of fasting lasts, you can consume water, as well as some calorie-free drinks.

Thus, it is similar to the 5:2 diet but stricter. Not eating anything for 24 hours twice a week is difficult for most people. However, the other days of the week, you can eat whatever you want, as long as it is healthy.

If 24 hours sounds impossible, then here is the good news. As per Pilon, this diet technique is flexible, so instead of the full 24 hours, 20 – 24 hours will also give you huge benefits.

Now, let's look at an example of an Eat Stop Eat IF routine:

- Let's say you eat normally until 7 pm on a Saturday, and then fast until 7 pm on Sunday. After that, you resume your regular eating schedule till Wednesday at 7 pm and eat approximately 2,000 kcal daily for women (2,500 for men), without fasting on any consecutive day. Finally, from 7 pm on Wednesday to 7 pm on Thursday, you have another fast and repeat the schedule.

You don't have to perform more than two fasts in one week. Pilon says that by doing even one fast per week, you can easily create a calorie deficit of 10%.

To burn fat and discover those lean, formed muscles more quickly, try to engage in some resistance or weight training when you are on Eat Stop Eat. Avoid cardio or other types of exhaustive exercises. As per Brad Pilon's Eat Stop Eat Quick Start Guide, a consistent workout routine of three to four times weekly, with two to four exercises per body part, three to five sets per exercise, and six to 15 repetitions per set is recommended. However, you don't have to exercise on the fasting days.

Advantages of Eat Stop Eat Method

- According to an article that was published in Obesity Reviews in 2011, executing an IF plan such as the Eat Stop Eat for 12 weeks, **causes weight loss** and retains more lean muscle mass.
- Other possible benefits, as stated by Pilon, are **reduced inflammation** and cellular cleansing.
- Lastly, practicing Eat Stop Eat may be **more straightforward** as compared to other diets in which you need to limit an entire food group, like carbohydrates or fats.

Disadvantages of Eat Stop Eat Method

- The Eat Stop Eat routine can **interfere with regular social interactions,** like meal plans with friends and family. So it is best done privately.

- The diet is **not recommended for pregnant women**, diabetics, and those with a history of eating disorders like binging.
- It can also **cause headaches and crankiness** in some people
- Finally, Eat Stop Eat **doesn't provide any specific recommendations regarding what to eat** during the non-fasting days. So, it's up to you to exercise self-control and decide what to eat. This can be challenging for those who struggle with weight issues and eating disorders.

Alternate Day Fasting

Alternate day fasting, also known as the "4/3 Intermittent Fasting" schedule or "Up-Day, Down-Day Diet," was created by James Johnson and is based on a simple philosophy: you fast one day, whether by eating 500 kcal or fewer or not eating at all, and the next day you eat as you usually do.

During this method, since you'll be fasting more frequently than you are on Eat Stop Eat or 5:2, the 4/3 IF routine can be slightly challenging to maintain.

As mentioned, there are two primary ways of executing the alternate day fasting diet.

- The first method is to alternate days of complete fasting – eating no solid food and consuming only unsweetened tea, coffee, or water – with eating normally.
- The second way is to alternate days of drastically reduced calorie intake with days of eating a regular diet. So on fasting days, you should consume one-fifth of your normal caloric intake, which is around 400 kcal for women (and 500 for men).
- If you cannot reduce by this much, you can increase your caloric intake to a maximum of 700 kcal if you are a woman (and to 875 if you're a man). For a 2,000 kcal daily diet for women and a 2,500 kcal daily diet for men, this comes out to be 25% – 35% of the regular intake.

For gaining muscle, exercising is recommended during the normal calorie days, since on low-calorie days you may find it difficult to work out, which might discourage you a little bit. Remember to eat enough protein and healthy fats so that you have tons of energy for your training sessions.

Advantages of Alternate Day Fasting

- Apart from helping you to lose weight, lengthen your lifespan, and decrease both your blood pressure, alternate day fasting also helps to **decrease the overall circulating cholesterol level.**
- According to research, this fasting method might help to **reduce the risk of developing certain types of cancers.**
- 4/3 Intermittent Fasting also has a psychological advantage over the other fasting techniques. **People tend to stick to this diet better** since, even though they become hungry on the fasting days, they know that they have a feasting day to look forward to the next day.

Disadvantages of Alternate Day Fasting

- Some participants might feel **exceedingly cranky and irritable** on the fasting days.
- When proper care is not taken, people may transform their normal calorie day into a lower calorie day. This can cause **severe calorie deficiency** leading to adverse health effects. Hence for this reason, if you choose to practice the 4/3 method, it is recommended to plan in advance the meals for the next day in order to

keep the level of calories within the desired safe range.

The Warrior Method

Introduced by Ori Hofmekler, the Warrior Diet involves eating a very small amount of food for 20 hours of the day ("undereating" phase), and then consuming the significant portion of your daily calories in the remaining four-hour "overeating" phase.

It is quite different from any other diet discussed so far. When starting the Warrior Diet, Hofmekler recommends following the three-stage plan – Detox, High Fat, and Concluding Fat Loss – to improve your body's ability to generate energy by efficiently utilizing body fat.

- The **Detox stage** lasts for one week and throughout this time you can eat small amounts of low-calorie food during the undereating phase such as raw fruits (apples, berries bananas, pineapples), raw vegetables (leafy greens, broccoli, mushrooms, carrots), vegetable juices, yogurt, cottage cheese, and hardboiled eggs. For the overeating window, you can have salad, beans, cooked veggies, rice, or oats.

- The second or the **High Fat stage** also lasts for one week. The meal plan for the 20-hour undereating phase remains the same. During the four hours of overeating, you must focus on fats and proteins, instead of grains or starches. So, you should eat salad, cooked vegetables, chicken or fish, and a handful of nuts.
- For the **Concluding Fat Loss stage**, you will have to alternate between high-carb and low-carb, high-protein meals. So you'll start with one to two days which are high in carbs, and follow it with one to two days that are low in carbs but high in proteins. Then repeat that cycle twice throughout the week.

You can continue eating the same foods during the undereating phase of the day. However, during the four-hour feasting window high-carb days, include oats, pasta, corn, potatoes, cooked vegetables, chicken or fish, and salad.

During the overeating part of your low-carb, high-protein days, have some salad with 8 to 16 ounces of chicken/fish, along with cooked, non-starchy vegetables. You can also have some fresh tropical fruits for dessert.

Once you have completed the first three weeks of the diet, you can switch to eating low-calorie meals for 20 hours and high-protein, nutrient-dense foods for four hours each day. Also, throughout the day, you can drink water and unsweetened coffee or tea.

To promote fat loss, incorporate strength and speed training into your routines.

Advantages of Warrior Method

- Practicing the Warrior Diet dramatically **improves your body's protein absorption** rate.
- Training during the undereating phase **enhances the rate of your muscle growth.**
- Since the overeating phase involves eating a large quantity of food in a short period of time, your body ends up **burning a lot of calories** digesting this food. This increases the rate of daily energy expenditure, ultimately causing weight loss.

Disadvantages of Warrior Method

- Since the eating time is reduced to a four-hour period, the Warrior Diet **may not suit everybody's lifestyle.**
- When starting the diet, you can **feel certain side effects** like dizziness, low energy,

hunger, irritability, low blood sugar, fainting, insomnia, and hormonal imbalance.

- If you've suffered from **eating disorders**, the Warrior Diet can lead to binge eating. This can cause feelings of regret and shame, and can negatively impact body image and mental health.
- The Warrior Diet is **not suitable for underweight people**, extreme athletes, women who are pregnant or nursing, and people with diseases like heart failure or certain cancers.

Fat Fasting

Fat Fasting is a form of high-fat, low-calorie diet in which you consume 1,000–1,250 kcal per day and 80–90% of these calories come from fat.

Since you are allowed to eat while following this technique, it is technically not a fast. However, it definitely mimics the fat reduction effects of a fast.

How? Well, in two ways. Firstly, Fat Fast is low in calories and high in fat. Due to this, it creates a calorie deficit that is essential for weight loss.

And secondly, this method of fasting moves your body into the fat burning process of ketosis.

Now, ketosis is a metabolic state in which your body generates heat by utilizing stored fats, instead of carbohydrates. As a result of this, your fat pockets slowly start decreasing. But, the ketosis condition can only be achieved when the level of glucose in your blood is less.

Fat Fasting does precisely that. By restricting foods that are high in proteins and carbs, this method lowers your blood glucose and triggers your body to get into the ketosis phase quickly.

Ketosis and Fat Fasting are components of the ketogenic diet. If you want to learn more about this, and about the ketogenic diet in general, such as why do it, how to do it, its benefits, disadvantages and much more, then do read my book on Ketogenic Diet.

Some precautions:

- Fat Fast should **only be practiced for 2–5 days**, as it lacks in many essential nutrients, including proteins, micronutrients, and fiber, all of which are essential for good health.
- Fat Fasting should only be done under the following three circumstances-
- If you have been unable to lose weight for more than 2-3 weeks, then you can use the

Fat Fast technique to **break your weight loss plateau.**

- **If you've had a "cheat day"** and would like to get back on track quickly the next day, you may try this method.
- Lastly, you should do Fat Fasting **only when your body is used to the ketogenic diet.** Otherwise, it can cause health problems, including keto flu. If you're not already keto-adapted, try following the ketogenic diet for about 3-4 weeks and then only use Fat Fast to break a weight loss plateau/get over your cheat day.

Here are the points you need to keep in mind to start Fat Fasting:

- Start by taking multivitamins to compensate for the missing micronutrients.
- Make sure you eat only those foods that are very high in fat, but low in proteins and carbohydrate content.
- Keep your total daily calorie consumption within 1,000–1,250 kcal, by eating 4-5 small meals per day, each about 200-250 kcal.
- Avoid doing any extensive exercise on the Fat Fast days. This does not mean you have

to be inactive. You can always include some light cardio (walking) or some strength training exercises at home like squats, press-ups, etc., but you must take it easy and stay away from intense workout.

What to Eat and What to Avoid?

Since Fat Fast is slightly different from the conventional methods of Intermittent Fasting, it has its own unique diet plan.

- When choosing the food items for your Fat Fast, make sure that they have a very high fat content. Some options are:
- Whole eggs
- Mayonnaise
- Oils: coconut oil, olive oil, and avocado oil
- High-fat fish and meats: sardines, salmon, and bacon
- Dairy: butter, heavy cream, cream cheese, and high-fat cheese like brie
- Nondairy products: coconut cream and full-fat coconut milk
- High-fat fruits and low-carb vegetables: olives, avocados, and non-starchy vegetables like spinach, kale, and zucchini cooked in fat.

- Nuts and nut butters: macadamia nuts, macadamia nut butter, etc.
- Drinks: water, coffee, tea, and sparkling water
- If you want to include chicken, add it in sparing amounts, only from a flavor perspective.
- Food items that are high in carbs and proteins but low in fat must be avoided during a Fat Fast.
- Confectionaries: cakes, pastries, sweets, biscuits, etc.
- Sweet drinks: energy drinks, juice, sweetened coffee, etc.
- Fruits and vegetables: avoid all, except the ones listed above
- Cereals and grains: oats, rice, bread, pasta, crackers, etc.
- Beans and pulses: black beans, lentils, butter beans, etc.
- Dairy foods: low-fat cheese, low-fat yogurt, skim milk, etc.
- Meats and fish: beef, lamb, chicken, cod, etc.

Advantages of Fat Fasting

- This method **helps to induce** yourself into **ketosis** quicker.
- During ketosis, your body is in a fat burning stage. By triggering ketosis fast, Fat Fasting helps to **lose a few pounds quickly.**
- It also helps to **break weight loss plateau.**
- Lastly, it also aids you in **getting back to ketosis after a cheat day.**

Disadvantages of Fat Fasting

- If you **haven't been following a ketogenic diet** before Fat Fasting, you can experience keto flu. The symptoms of keto flu are headaches, diarrhea, nausea, constipation, fatigue, dizziness, muscle cramps, and stomach pains.
- Lack of proteins, carbs, fibers, and micronutrients in your diet can cause **nutrient deficiencies** if you practice Fat Fast for more than five days
- A longer duration of Fat Fasting may also put you at a **risk of muscle wasting** due to the lack of calories and proteins in the diet. Muscle wasting occurs when the body breaks down your muscle fibers to meet its protein

and energy needs, which your diet fails to provide.

- **People who have heart disease or diabetes** or are taking medications should consult their doctors before beginning a Fat Fast.
- This technique is also **not recommended for women who are pregnant or breastfeeding.**
- Fat Fasting can cause a **significant increase in cholesterol levels.** So if you are someone who is a cholesterol hyper-responder, avoid this method.

Fasting Mimicking Diet

The Fasting Mimicking Diet or FMD was developed by Dr. Valter Longo, an Italian biologist, and researcher.

Fast Mimicking is a form of modified fasting, in which instead of completely abstaining from food like in a traditional fasting practice, you still take in a little amount of food in such a way that you reap the therapeutic benefits and advantages that come with doing a fast.

In other words, the Fasting Mimicking Diet, like its name implies, mimics fasting.

FMD involves eating low protein, moderate carb, moderate fat foods. It generally lasts for about five days a month, and the number of months depends on the person concerned.

To prepare yourself for the five-day FMD, it is recommended that you start following a low protein diet (0.36 grams of protein per pound of your body weight) per day for one week. This protein should come from fish and vegetables. Along with that, have multivitamin and omega-3 supplement at least twice during this preparatory week.

Once you have done this, here is how the next five days will be like:

Day 1: 56% fat, 34% carbs, 10% protein

During day one, you can eat approximately 1,100 kcal, 500 from healthy fats and 500 from complex carbohydrates. Also include about 25 grams of plant-based protein (which is approximately 100 kcal), such as nuts.

Day 2-5: 44% fat, 47% carbs, 9% protein

For the remaining four days, you are required to further reduce the calorie consumption to only 800 kcal per day. 400 kcal will be from complex carbohydrates and 400 from healthy fats.

Day 6: Transition day

For 24 hours following the end of the five-day FMD, you should follow a diet comprised of complex carbohydrates. This includes rice, vegetables, fruit, etc. You should minimize the consumption of meat, fish, saturated fats, cheese, pastries, and milk.

After day 6, you can return to a regular eating schedule.

Doing intense workout isn't recommend during this five-day fasting period. Instead, you can incorporate light exercises, like walking or yoga, to keep your body active.

Advantages of Fasting Mimicking Diet

By reducing calories, Fasting Mimicking essentially "tricks" your body into believing that it is in fasting state. As a result, FMD has all the benefits that are commonly associated with Intermittent Fasting.

Disadvantages of Fasting Mimicking Diet

- The Fasting Mimicking Diet program is rich in nuts. So **if you have nut allergy**, FMD is not for you.

- This method is also not recommended for those who are **underweight** or malnourished.
- **Pregnant or breastfeeding women** must avoid FMD.
- **People on medications** or those who have kidney or heart disease should follow this diet under their doctor's supervision.
- Lastly, if you have **eating disorders,** FMD might not be appropriate for you.

I want you to believe that from here on only the best of health awaits you.

Overcoming diabetes, hypertension, and obesity is no more beyond your reach. Many people all over the world are successfully taking control of their health with the help of Intermittent Fasting, and so can you.

The techniques I have discussed in this chapter are some of the most widely practiced ones. So do try them. They work time and time again. I and many others are a true testament to the contributions of these methods toward weight loss and everlasting health.

Chapter 6

Intermittent Fasting to Lose Weight

The weight loss benefits of any Intermittent Fasting plan are obvious – in addition to assisting with metabolism, the diet also helps to curb your appetite, which means you eat less.

With IF, it is essential to understand that it is possible to gain weight instead of losing if your diet is not appropriate. To see fruitful results, you must implement a dietary schedule which ensures that you achieve a caloric deficit, while still providing your body with the essential nutrients it relies on daily to perform all the functions that are crucial to your own survival.

Different types of meal plans have been suggested for those who are looking to lose weight through Intermittent Fasting. But in the end, it is up to you to choose a diet routine that suits you the most. You will have to take yourself into account – consider how much weight you want to lose, and any particular health conditions that you may be suffering from.

In the previous chapter, as part of our second step to mastering IF, we have already discussed the various options out there that you can select from.

Most people find that the standard 16/8 IF program to be ideal for them. Though some are able to follow the program through the entire week, you can vary the number of days as per your convenience.

However, in the end, you will essentially have to listen to your own body – if you feel that you are starving yourself too much, adjust your plan in order to make up for the excessive reduction in your daily caloric consumption.

On the contrary, if you find that you are not losing weight, it might be a good idea to have a look at your calorie balance – how much calories are you consuming and how much are you burning through physical activity?

Now that you understand the basics of Intermittent Fasting, how it affects women differently than male fasters, and how to choose the best personalized fasting schedule to meet your needs, keep reading to learn the next steps that must be executed to ensure personal success with Intermittent Fasting!

Step Three: Fit Bodies Are Made In The Kitchen

Adventure can be fun, but new habits and routines rarely run smoothly or even get off of the ground without some planning and preparation.

This is particularly true for women thanks to the many biological, hormonal, genetic, and environmental factors that can affect female participants from seeing the positive results they hope for with Intermittent Fasting.

There are ways to counteract these issues when they come up, and in some cases, even help prevent them from interfering with your progress.

Stock Your Kitchen To Support An Intermittent Fasting Routine

Intermittent Fasting is not just about avoiding food. It is also about choosing the right types and amounts of food to be consumed during feeding, feasting or refueling windows (though I tend to incline more toward refueling, you can choose whichever term you prefer the most).

It is during these windows the fasters can focus on the type of diet they want to pair with their Intermittent Fasting plan to get the most out of their new health and wellness-inspired lifestyle.

However, it is essential to remember that you do not have to change your eating habits if you are content with your current dietary program or if you are required to stick to a specific type of food consumption due to existing health concerns.

One of the best parts about Intermittent Fasting and something that is continuously praised and spoken of in health circles, is its ability to be adapted to any existing diet. This means that those with diet-related health conditions such as gluten intolerance, lactose intolerance, or insulin dependency can take part in fasting as a health enhancement tool without threatening their physical health or making matters worse.

There are plenty of diets that can be used alongside Intermittent Fasting to create a well-rounded and thorough wellness program, but most experts recommend adopting a low carbohydrate and high protein diet.

Foods that are rich in carbohydrates are typically high in sugar as well, and carbs break down into glucose more quickly than other food groups. On the other side of the spectrum, foods that have a high protein content take longer to digest. Thus eating protein makes the person feel fuller for more extended periods of time. Also, protein-rich meals are low in fats and carbohydrates, which makes them less likely to be broken down to be stored as fat deposits instead of being burned off.

Regardless of the diet you choose, some steps and actions can be taken to ensure that you have all the necessary food items in your pantry to easily adjust to a healthy lifestyle with Intermittent Fasting. Some of these actions include:

- Switching out all processed fats like margarine for healthier cooking oils like coconut oil or olive oil.
- Making the switch from refined sugars and sweeteners for healthy alternatives like agave nectar or natural and local honey.
- Removing all junk food, sugary drinks, and fatty desserts that could damage forward progress via overconsumption of calories.
- Replace unhealthy snack options with healthier alternatives like low-carb condiments, snack foods, and treats to satisfy a sweet tooth without disturbing your diet or wellness plan.
- Fill your cookbooks with low-carb recipes that are as full of flavor as they are with health benefits.
- Make sure to find a good collection of healthy snack and dessert recipes that can be made quickly to help you on nights when snacking and binging are threatening to throw you off your game.

Basically, when it comes to the kitchen: out with the fatty, carb-filled and sugary foods, and in with the organic, local and higher quality meats and produce that can enhance the health benefits of an Intermittent Fasting lifestyle.

Example Meal Plan For Weight Loss With Intermittent Fasting

If you do a quick Google search for weight loss plans that work in conjunction with IF, you'll be surprised at the sheer number of variations available out there. This can make the entire process very challenging, and a far cry from the fun and exciting journey that Intermittent Fasting can be.

Many of the weight loss plans available can be useful if you stick to the plan and ensure your body is provided with an adequate amount of exercise on a daily basis.

Below, I will introduce you to an example of an excellent Intermittent Fasting diet plan that you can use if you're finding it hard to choose one by yourself. It has a very basic "framework" that you can follow and adjust according to your own preferences and requirements.

But before we look at the example, there is one thing that you should note.

- Do not expect everything to go smoothly the first time around. On the first few days, know that situations can be rather tricky. This is especially true if you are used to eating continuously during the day – which is a widespread problem among people who have a considerable amount of weight to lose.
- Be patient in the beginning – with yourself and with the results you want to achieve through your diet plan. After a week or two, if you do not see the desired outcome, then make a few adjustments to your diet plan and IF program so that those are in sync with your goals.

With the diet plan example that I'm about to share with you, I want you to get into a habit of skipping breakfast. You will only have a window of six to eight hours, where you will consume food every day. Since you are aiming to lose weight, skipping out on breakfast will allow your body to utilize its own fat reserves in order to generate energy.

You will then have your first meal at 3 pm in the afternoon, your second meal at around 6 pm and then finish off the day with a final dinner at around 10 pm.

Keep the first two meals light. This way, you won't turn off your body's automatic fat burning mechanisms. The final and last meal, however, can be a little heavier on the calorie side.

I personally recommend that the first two meals of your day should be a maximum of 400 kcal each. Ensure that there is an ample supply of protein in these meals. Don't skim on vegetables and fruits – include them as they are good for you.

Here are some examples of small and light dishes that you can experiment with for your first two meals (at 3 pm and 6 pm):

- Add some almonds and a couple of berries into a cup of Greek yogurt.
- Have some cottage cheese with a couple of almonds.
- Add one tablespoon of olive oil to a can of tuna, and enjoy your meal with an apple.
- Use two whole eggs to make yourself an omelet. Have this meal with some delicious berries.
- If you're in the mood to eat a meatier meal, then cook up a chicken breast and enjoy it with some green salad. You can add half avocado to the meal, as well as an apple.

- For those who are in a hurry and would like to drink something instead, mixing a cup of unsweetened almond milk with about 40 grams of whey protein powder is a perfect option. You can have some fruit with this, as well as about 20 grams of almonds.

When it comes to the third item of the day – this is when you should enter the full chef-mode and prepare yourself something healthy and delicious. There are a lot of different healthy meals that you can choose to fill the gap at 10 pm. It is better to limit the last meal of the day to around 800 kcal, but you can push it up to about 1000 kcal if you wish.

During the last meal, it is essential to balance fats and protein perfectly to avoid weight gain or other potential side-effects from your diet plan.

- If you are opting for lean meat (to supply your body with quality protein), then you can have more healthy types of fats in your meal.
- If, on the other side, you decide to opt for a fattier kind of meal, let's say a piece of fatty steak, then you should limit how much added fats you put into your dish.

To help you prepare your third and final meal of the day, here are three examples of recipes that are nutritious and will give you that final amount of calories you need during your eating window:

- Cook up a chicken breast and serve it with some potato wedges and a variety of vegetables.
- Serve some brown rice with vegetables and a chicken breast. Try to use a small amount of coconut oil for cooking both the rice and the chicken.
- Instead, if you're in the mood for having some beef, then have a steak with some vegetables. You can also serve this up with a sweet potato. Add a little bit of cinnamon to the sweet potato for additional flavor.

Different foods can have vastly varied effects on your hunger, hormones, and the number of calories you burn. Even though you are free to experiment with the food items you consume during each meal, always remember your end goal, which is to lose weight and become a healthier person.

Step Four: Be Prepared To Exercise Before You Jump Right In!

Regular exercise is one of the critical aspects of maintaining a healthy figure and lifestyle. However, starting an Intermittent Fasting routine can take a toll on the body in the early days.

Still, it is often recommended that as a new faster, you should not wholly stop exercising until you see how your body responds. If fatigue, muscle weakness, and other negative side effects become apparent, you can either reduce the intensity of your workout or at least make sure that you do not push yourself beyond your tolerance levels.

Exercising With Intermittent Fasting

Ask anyone who has had successful results with any type of dieting program in the past – and they will tell you that exercise was a crucial part of their weight loss routine. The primary idea behind any kind of diet that aims to help you reduce the unwanted body fat is to create a caloric deficit.

Thus, when you include a weight loss diet plan along with Intermittent Fasting, you should ensure that you implement an appropriate exercise program as well.

Some people get concerned when told to exercise while following an IF program. However, once your body is used to this new eating style, you will notice that it becomes easier and easier to work out. Also, there are a variety of supplements that you can take to boost your endurance and stamina and to give you that extra dose of energy to get past a training session, even while you are fasting.

Here is a little-known secret that many people do not realize in terms of exercising and IF. The fat burning mechanisms of the human body is regulated by what is known as the Sympathetic Nervous System. This system is also called the SNS for short. When the system activates, it means your body starts to burn fat.

There are two essential elements that cause the SNS system to activate – a lack of food in your body and exercise. When you decide to give your body a dose of both, the SNS gets fully triggered. This activation of SNS increases the efficiency of fat burning processes in the body, thereby leading to weight loss.

But this isn't the only reason why a reduction in calorie intake can improve the efficiency of your workout.

Take this into account as well – if you eat before your exercise program, then there is a chance that the consumed food may lead to issues with your general performance during the training.

It has been found that consumption of food in any form – be it a shake, an energy bar, or an actual meal – causes your blood glucose levels to spike while you are exercising. Sure, this will give you some energy to kickstart that tough routine you're about to begin – but, once this spike is over, your blood glucose levels will quickly decline, and you will basically experience a "crash." What this indicates is that your body will run out of energy and you will feel fatigued, which will ultimately lead to poor muscle performance.

There are, however, some publications that say this is a myth – still, this is something that you should consider when it comes to Intermittent Fasting!

In a nutshell, these are some of the benefits that you can reap by integrating a good workout program into your IF plan.

- Due to the positive impact of exercise on your body, while it is in a fasting state, you can turn back what is known as the "biological clock" in your brain, as well as your muscles.

- The concentration of Human Growth Hormone or HGH produced by your body will increase.
- The body composition will also significantly improve, due to a reduction in body fat percentage, along with an increase in lean muscle mass.
- Along with that, you'll see an improvement in cognitive functions, and problems like brain fog will start to disappear.
- Your testosterone levels are likely to rise as well, which can be especially beneficial for older men who are experiencing a natural decline in the level of circulating testosterone within their bodies.

As per experts and long-time fasting participants, you must exercise when your body seems to have the most energy to spend on physical activities. Also, the workout routine must not leave you fatigued during work, school, and other daily obligations or interfere with the course of your everyday life.

Therefore, you must engage in physical activities that are just enough to get the heart pumping and the body moving, such as taking a small walk, doing some stretching exercises or light cardio, and practicing yoga.

However, there are a few exceptions that I must warn you about.

- On days when you feel to do some intense workout as part of your exercise routine, it is crucial to eat something within the first 30 minutes after completing the training. Fast-assimilating proteins such as whey protein is an option.
- Even after trying a couple of times, if you find that you're unable to exercise on an empty stomach, have some fruit immediately prior to the workout. Since you can easily burn it during the exercise, it won't impair insulin sensitivity and will also provide some initial fuel to help kickstart your training routine.

Get A Professional Opinion To Guarantee Health & Safety

The best advice to take when it comes to diets, fitness, and fasting is that from a healthcare professional, preferably a personal physician who is already familiar with your medical history and current health status.

If a personal physician cannot be involved, a dietician or nutritionist can provide medical information about potential risks and offer valuable advice on how to derive the maximize benefits from an Intermittent Fasting plan.

Intermittent Fasting Tip: Keep A Record Of Your Personal Experience

It is always better to stay alert and take some safety precautions when it comes to making significant lifestyle changes that could potentially affect or bring attention to the existing health conditions.

Keeping a health diary or some record of how you are feeling as you start your personal Intermittent Fasting plan can be helpful for a number of reasons including:

- Creating a list of symptoms, when they started, how long they lasted and their intensity
- Providing a reliable account of happenings, events, obstacles and other circumstances that may have affected your Intermittent Fasting schedule
- Serving as a reminder of all the progress that has been made throughout your IF journey on days where it may be challenging to stay determined and focused on your health goals

A personal journal will also come in handy when the time comes to make changes to your personalized fasting schedule in order to

- minimize any side effects
- increase the challenge when the body has adapted to the current plan and has slowed or ceased forward progress.

This can happen over time, making it seem as though Intermittent Fasting has become ineffective. The truth is that like with any diet or fitness program, the body learns to adjust to the fasting process and can become immune to its more dynamic effects like weight loss and fat burning.

For those who have attained their health goals, there may not be a need to intensify your personalized IF routine as long as you feel fit and all the positive progress you made do not start reversing.

It's all a matter of personal preference and planning. Not everyone will need to make major changes to their fasting plan, but having a record of your experiences will surely help along the line.

It doesn't need to be each day. Only when the symptoms or events are noteworthy like unusual hunger pangs or a severe headache that just wouldn't seem to go away, you can write it down in your journal to serve as a future reference.

Your health diary should also include the positive events, such as hitting a certain goal, discovering a new recipe that works within your preferred diet or setting new goals after progress has been made, for that extra motivation.

Step Five: Schedule Your First Fasting Plan

Taking the first step of any journey is a fascinating, confusing and exciting action, and IF is no exception.

The good news is that with the help of this guide, and by

- collecting all the necessary information,
- writing down your goals and motivations,
- choosing the right fasting schedule as per your needs,
- stocking your kitchen with healthy staples, and
- taking control of your daily fitness routine to help with adjusting to the new fasting and feeding windows,

you have already begun setting yourself up for success on your personal Intermittent Fasting journey.

Plan Out More Than Just One Week At A Time

One of the best ways to achieve success before you even start fasting is to plan out three to four weeks of fasting and feeding windows at a time.

Many find that having a calendar, chart, or other kinds of visual representation of their Intermittent Fasting routine helps with things like:

- Keeping track of their fasting and feeding days
- Keeping track of progress made and when goals are scheduled
- Making plans with friends and family around their IF schedule or knowing how to prepare or adjust their routine in order to fully enjoy the events and meetings with the people they love
- Planning meals, making grocery lists and scheduling fitness windows

Getting into this habit of preparing your fasting routine in three to four-week blocks ahead of time, by creating a schedule that can be seen and referenced whenever the need arises, will help you to stay focused and dedicated to your Intermittent Fasting schedule in the long-run.

Choosing The Best Day To Start A New Intermittent Fasting Routine

The best day to start any new change that can have an effect on both the physical and mental functions in your body is a day where your schedule is at its most relaxed and you have at least one day (preferably two days) to rest following it.

The main reason for this is that no one person knows for sure how their body is going to react to the fasting plan they have chosen, particularly if this is their first time ever trying Intermittent Fasting or they haven't taken the time to ease themselves into their new fasting plan.

Starting a fasting plan on a demanding day at work or any other day that requires an individual to be at their physical and mental peak performance is not recommended as fatigue, nausea, hunger, and dehydration are some of the most common side effects reported on the first day of an IF routine.

However, it must also be mentioned that not everyone experiences adverse effects on the first day. Sometimes it can take up to a week for the body to respond to the changes. By that time, fasting becomes a regular part of the person's daily routine.

This is why having at least a couple of days off after one's first fasting window (especially if it is a longer window or happening at the start of a dietary change) is recommended, particularly for those who are new to Intermittent Fasting.

Many people like to start their IF schedules on a three-day weekend or spring break. Others stay true to the spiritual origins of fasting and start their fasting routine during holy times such as Lent or Ramadan.

It all comes down to personal preference. Just make sure to take the time and lay out a plan before just diving in, or you'll be starting out at a disadvantage.

What To Expect In The First Week On A New Intermittent Fasting Schedule

For those new to Intermittent Fasting, the first week can be the most worrisome and challenging.

Knowing what to look out for and how to overcome the obstacles that develop in the early days of a new Intermittent Fasting routine can help make the transition painless and enjoyable.

Here are some of the symptoms that you can expect in the first week of your IF schedule:

- At first, you will **feel really hungry**. But know that it is entirely normal. In order to make your fasting process significantly easier, eat a high-protein snack before you start the fast, such as fish, chicken, cottage cheese, egg, oats, quinoa, lentils, almonds, peanuts, etc.
- During the first two days, you may experience a few side effects like **bad breath, nausea, dizziness, and headaches.** These are just the signs of your body trying to flush out the toxins.
- Between days three and seven, **your skin might feel a little oily,** leading to acne breakouts. However, after the first week, the skin will get clearer.
- You can also experience **muscle weakness, constipation, and other digestive complications.**
- You may find that you are **easily getting distracted** or having difficulty in gaining or maintaining focus
- Another effect many women specifically report in their first week of a new fasting routine (between the first three and five days on their fast schedule) is some **trouble in falling asleep.**

The good news is that, after the first week is over, almost everybody practicing Intermittent Fasting as part of their daily lives, fall asleep quickly. It has also been seen that participants experience deeper periods of sleep the more they stick with their personalized fasting plan.

Intermittent Fasting Tip: Drink More Water Than Before

Dehydration is one of the most common side effects reported by both men and women during their Intermittent Fasting routine.

The main reason for this is that water weight is the first to go when fasting and fat burning processes take over. Thus the body requires more hydration than before in order to comfortably function and perform.

Any adverse effects related to dehydration can be easily diminished or even avoided by simply ensuring you're consuming six to eight glasses of water a day.

- Hunger pangs are typical in the first week of IF. But most of the times they can be attributed to thirst and dehydration, rather than the lack of food consumption.

So, do pay attention the next time you feel hungry while fasting. Drink some water first. If you still feel starving, then only break your fast and eat something.

Drinking plenty of water during the day and especially during the fasting windows is also the best way to combat all the six issues new fasters face during the first week of their Intermittent Fasting.

Along with that, eating enough calories during the feeding windows and giving your the body time to adapt to a fluctuating eating and fasting schedule also aid in preventing the symptoms of dehydration from interfering with your personal health progress.

Step Six: Know How To Continue Your Fast

Sustaining any fast can be a tough thing to do. Because of the discomfort people go through during the first few days of their IF schedule, they feel the conditions will never get better and thus they give up.

Unless you are suffering from an actual medical issue that can potentially become worse during the fast, breaking the fast early will not benefit your body in any way. You are not going to see any health benefits if you continue breaking your fasts early and then eat a ton of extra food.

To ensure that you continue your fast and not break out of it early, here are some things you can do.

- **Set the right objectives:** Before getting started on a fast, take time to remind yourself of the reasons you are doing the fast in the first place. Is it for health reasons or religious reasons or just to lose weight?

Setting your objectives ahead of time will help you to stay focused when things get tough.

- **Inform someone about your fasting:** Tell a friend or a family member that you are going to embark on an Intermittent Fasting routine to lose weight and to become healthy.

This way, you will have someone to hold you accountable, which can make a ton of difference. You'll notice that by making the commitment and having someone to monitor you, it will be hard for you to break your fast or quit it altogether.

- **Maintain a journal:** I have already discussed why you should maintain a health diary or journal.

In addition to those benefits, logging and journaling can also help you to sustain your fast.

Write down your daily objectives, what you have eaten during the day, and how you are feeling during the fasting. You might not notice it at first, but writing down everything in your journal can give you a good glimpse of how your body is becoming fit. And when you see this, it will definitely motivate you to continue with your fast.

Intermittent Fasting involves adjusting to a new lifestyle that promotes overall health and wellness.

For your quick reference, I'll summarize the steps we have discussed in this chapter.

Once you have chosen your preferred Intermittent Fasting method to meet your personal health goals, the next step is to take the information you have gathered and follow these steps:

- Make a list of everything you will need to stock your kitchen before your first official Intermittent Fasting window.
- Choose a day to start your Intermittent Fasting plan.
- Set your personalized schedule from there for at least the next three to four weeks. This will help with meal planning, scheduling events with friends and family, grocery budgeting, and so much more!

- Keep exercising.
- Maintain a health journal.
- If you ever feel like giving up, you know what to do!

Now, that it's all planned out, prepare yourself to get started and take the plunge toward your long-term health and happiness!

Chapter 7

Intermittent Fasting in Our Life

We all know that we need to eat healthier food. We also know that we need to limit how much soda, juice, processed foods, and sugars we consume. However, even though we are aware of all these things, it doesn't mean that it is as easy to follow.

- The first thing we should have a look at is the quantity of food we are eating. The number of calories that each individual needs, varies from person to person and depends on various factors such as genetics, activity level, overall health, height, age, and gender.

However, the benchmark number that is used on food labels is about 2,000 kcal each day. This number is already fairly high for those who live a sedentary life. Additionally, it is possible to eat 2,000 kcal (or more) in just one sitting if you go out to eat or order food in. While eating out regularly pushes us past our calorie limits, it is also possible to eat more when you are at home.

Hence, it is vital that you are aware of your eating patterns. Rather than eating something just because it tastes good or because you are bored, tired, or sad, you have to learn to consume only those items that you need to function.

- The time of day that we eat can matter as well. Most of us live a busy lifestyle, so we don't have the time to sit down and eat well-balanced meals. Instead, we eat on the go, usually at some place that is unhealthy, or eat directly at night when our metabolisms are slower.
- Additionally, many of us spend our free time sitting on the couch and eating unhealthy snack foods while watching television. Sometimes, food is so abundant that we eat non-stop.

Therefore, the two primary reasons due to which you are unable to lose weight are consuming unhealthy food or sources of glucose and the habit of constantly eating.

When you go on an Intermittent Fast, you force the body to stop relying on a constant source of glucose to fuel it. Since you go so long without eating, your body has to look for some form of fuel to help it function. Thus it resorts to burning the stored glycogen of the body, or the stored body fat.

Intermittent Fasting is all about adding short fasts into your daily life, with a goal to minimize the number of calories you consume in a day. Just by doing these short-term fasts each day, your hormones will be stimulated, you will burn the extra fat stored in your body, cut out calories, and lose weight faster than ever before.

You must have heard about the three most popular forms of diet in the health and fitness world – paleo, vegan, and keto.

Just like IF, all these are complete lifestyle changes rather than short-term weight loss strategies.

Due to these similarities and their overall health benefits, many fitness enthusiasts combine Intermittent Fasting with one of the three forms of dieting to obtain even better results.

Let's discuss about each of these three combinations and also the effect IF has on your hormones.

Intermittent Fasting &How It Affects Your Hormones

The body fat that you carry around is simply the way your body stores any unused energy or calories that you take in via food. When you go through a period of not eating anything, your body experiences changes that help it to access the stored energy better.

During fasting, your hormone levels get affected due to which a few changes occur in your metabolism. The hormones that get influenced are:

- **Norepinephrine:** The nervous system sends this hormone to your stored fat cells. This hormone causes the fat cells to break down into free fatty acids. The body then takes these fatty acids and uses them to generate energy.
- **HGH or human growth hormone:** Levels of the HGH hormone can increase like crazy during Intermittent Fasting. This hormone can help boost the efficiency of many processes in the body, including muscle gain and fat loss.
- **Insulin:** When you eat any food, your insulin increases. But when you go on a fast, your insulin levels decrease quite a bit. Lower levels of insulin in the body help to burn more fat.

Despite what proponents of five to six meals each day say, going on these short-term fasts can actually help in increasing the amount of fat that you can burn during the day. In fact, two studies found that fasting for a 48-hour time period can help boost your metabolism by up to 14 percent.

The fantastic thing about Intermittent Fasting is that it affects your hormones in a natural way. As long as your fasting period doesn't last for more than 48 hours, IF is not going to cause any harm to the body.

Instead, Intermittent Fasting will positively affect your hormones, so they behave in a way that is beneficial to you. Your body will be in a better position to regulate the insulin levels, keep your metabolism moving fast, and even help you feel less hungry throughout the day.

However, if you go for a fasting period that is too long, such as a 72-hour fast, it can actually suppress the hormones and ultimately, your metabolism.

So be careful about this one. Stick with the short-term fasts to enhance your metabolic activities and get the most out of fasting.

Intermittent Fasting & Paleo Diet

What is a paleo diet?

A paleo diet typically includes eating unprocessed, whole animal & plant foods such as nuts, meat, seeds, fish, fruits, eggs, and vegetables — foods that in the past could be obtained by hunting and gathering.

The diet restricts the consumption of processed foods, legumes, grains, sugar, and dairy products.

Contrary to most diets, the paleo diet doesn't involve the practice of counting calories. Rather, it restricts some food groups that are the primary sources of calories.

Other names for the paleo diet include caveman diet, hunter-gatherer diet, Paleolithic diet, and the Stone Age diet.

Purpose

The aim of following a paleo diet is to return to a way of eating that's more similar to what early humans ate.

The principle behind the diet is based on an idea known as the "discordance hypothesis" according to which the human body does not genetically match the current diet that has emerged with the modern farming practices.

Farming changed the eating habits of the people and established dairy, legumes, and grains as the additional staples in the human diet. The relatively late and rapid change in the food, according to the hypothesis, outpaced the body's ability to adapt to it. This mismatch is believed to be one of the contributing factors leading to the prevalence of diabetes, obesity, and heart disease today.

Why follow a paleo diet?

You may choose to follow a paleo diet for the following reasons:

- To initially lose weight, and then eventually maintain the healthy weight achieved
- Better appetite management
- Improved glucose tolerance
- Lower triglycerides
- Better blood pressure control

What to eat as part of a paleo diet?

Following food items can be present in your paleo diet:

- Fruits
- Vegetables
- Fish, particularly those that are rich in omega-3 fatty acids, such as salmon, mackerel and tuna
- Lean meats, especially from grass-fed animals or wild game
- Nuts and seeds
- Oils such as olive oil or walnut oil

What foods to avoid?

To practice the paleo diet, eliminate these food items from your meals:

- Legumes, such as lentils, beans, peanuts, and peas
- Grains, such as wheat, oats, and barley
- Refined sugar
- Dairy products
- Potatoes
- Salt
- Highly processed foods in general

A Sample Paleo Menu

If you want to try out the paleo diet, here is a sample menu. Feel free to adjust it as per your preferences.

Monday

- Breakfast: Eggs, vegetables cooked in coconut oil, along with one fruit.
- Lunch: Salad with olive oil, chicken, and a handful of nuts.
- Dinner: Fish, vegetables, and some salsa.

Tuesday

- Breakfast: Bacon, eggs, and a fruit.

- Lunch: Leftover dinner from the night before.
- Dinner: Vegetables and salmon fried in butter.

Wednesday

- Breakfast: Meat along with vegetables (leftovers from the night before).
- Lunch: Sandwich with lettuce leaves, meat, and fresh veggies.
- Dinner: Ground beef with veggies and some berries.

Thursday

- Breakfast: Eggs and one piece of fruit.
- Lunch: A handful of nuts and leftover dinner from the night before.
- Dinner: Fried pork and vegetables.

Friday

- Breakfast: Eggs, vegetables cooked in coconut oil.
- Lunch: A handful of nuts, chicken, and salad with olive oil
- Dinner: Steak, along with vegetables and sweet potatoes.

Saturday

- Breakfast: Bacon and eggs with one piece of fruit.
- Lunch: Leftover steak and vegetable dinner from the night before.
- Dinner: Baked salmon along with vegetables and avocado.

Sunday

- Breakfast: Meat along with the vegetables left from the night before
- Lunch: Sandwich with a lettuce leaf, fresh veggies, and meat..
- Dinner: Grilled chicken wings along with vegetables and salsa.

The diet also emphasizes on drinking plenty of water and being physically active every day.

Why combine IF and paleo diet?

Paleo diet and Intermittent Fasting work so well together.

And combining them is probably the most natural way to eat. If you want to follow paleo, why not follow it exactly like our ancestors?

Back in the Stone Age, early men would eat like in a paleo diet, and then that would be followed a fasting period.

This was because, during the day, they would move around from one place to another, hunting and collecting food. They wouldn't sit down to eat. They sometimes might snack on nuts or fruit or that they gathered. But, it was only in the evening that they would eat a large meal comprising of meat and vegetables.

Downsides to combining paleo and IF

There are two significant disadvantages of this combination.

- If you are used to unhealthy diet and carb-heavy breakfast, then changing to paleo and IF will be very difficult. In such a case, you must first start with a gradual change to healthy paleo living and then add fasting to the mix.
- Eating enough healthy and nutrient dense food within a short period daily can be tough for some people, especially those who are used to eating junk food.

Intermittent Fasting & Vegan Diet

When you look at the fundamental principles of Intermittent Fasting and the fundamental principles of veganism, you may find that these two lifestyles actually share quite a bit in common. While IF acts as a guideline for **when** you can eat, veganism lays down a framework for **what** you can eat. How you choose to incorporate each of these principles into your life really comes down to personal preference.

Similarities

Both intermittent fasters and vegans often come from a place of caring for their health and wanting to do what is best for their bodies, and these desires are reflected in the shared principles between these two lifestyles.

Lifestyle, Not a Diet -

We hear it all the time - **this is a lifestyle, not a diet -** but in the case of both Intermittent Fasting and veganism, it really is the truth.

A diet will often come with a grocery list, a meal plan, a set of instructions, and an overall restrictive approach to eating. Lifestyles, on the other hand, are flexible and focus instead on the ways in which this new way of eating can work for you.

Intermittent Fasting and veganism simply provide frameworks to guide you down the right path and leave plenty of room for you to play around with the variations, so that you can find a method that suits your current lifestyle the most.

Various Beliefs -

With both of these being lifestyles rather than diets, IF and veganism are built on some pretty deep-rooted beliefs, but these beliefs often vary from one person to the next.

Those who are strong supporters of Intermittent Fasting may believe in the physical health benefits, the mental health benefits, or the religious and spiritual reasons. Those who stand behind veganism may do it for the animals, the environment, or their own well-being.

However, what makes both Intermittent Fasting and veganism so widespread is the fact that they are flexible and all-encompassing. No matter what you believe in at your core, certain aspects of these lifestyles can and will resonate with you to some degree.

Importance of Exercise -

As with any healthy lifestyle, engaging in some form of physical activity on a regular basis is just as important as eating a well-balanced diet. Being conscious of what you are putting into your body often goes hand in hand with paying attention to how you are moving your body, and that is indeed the case with these lifestyles.

Sure, the IF community may lean more toward weight lifting and extreme sports while the vegan community may promote yoga and long-distance running, but these are of course just stereotypes and generalizations. At the end of the day, exercise is exercise, and both fasting and veganism promote an all-around healthy lifestyle, inclusive of both physical and mental health.

Food Quality -

Whether you're a hardcore faster or a hardcore vegan, chances are you probably care about the type of foods you are putting in your body.

What makes these lifestyles realistic and sustainable for most people is that they preach eating whole, nutrient-dense foods, and staying away from processed junk. The recommended breakdown of protein, carbohydrates, and fats may differ from one source to the next, but a diet consisting of mainly natural, high-quality foods is something that everyone can agree on. This can then lead to greater nutritional awareness and may even help eliminate nutrient deficiencies.

The Compound Benefits -

Intermittent Fasting and veganism each provide tremendous results on their own, and when combined, the benefits of these two lifestyles fuse together effortlessly.

The combination of IF and a whole food plant-based diet can actually reduce your risk of disease more than either approach ever could on its own, partly because combining the teachings of these two methods results in a highly anti-inflammatory way of eating. And this is just one of the many ways that incorporating Intermittent Fasting into your vegan lifestyle can be beneficial.

Reduced Inflammation -

People typically experience inflammation when the body is trying to heal itself. This means that inflammation in itself is not a bad thing, but when it remains untreated for a long duration of time, it can cause negative health outcomes.

Both Intermittent Fasting and veganism significantly reduce inflammation in the body due to calorie restriction and consumption of dietary fiber, respectively. Calorie restriction leads to autophagy, ketogenesis, and insulin sensitivity, all of which reduce inflammation.

Similarly, a diet rich in fiber reduces inflammation, possibly due to plant chemicals called phytonutrients found in fiber-rich fruits and vegetables. Additional anti-inflammatory vegan foods include leafy greens, sweet potatoes, blueberries, nuts and seeds, soy products, whole grains, turmeric, and garlic.

Weight Loss -

Individuals turn to IF and veganism for a variety of reasons, and weight loss is often the number one. This is actually quite interesting because neither of these lifestyles primarily market themselves to the weight loss community, but people are intrigued by the results that they see in other people.

When it comes down to it, weight loss is a simple equation of calories in versus calories out, and Intermittent Fasting and veganism make it easier to maintain a calorie deficit. By limiting the time in which you eat to say an 8-hour eating window and consuming a diet built around whole, plant-based foods, people naturally tend to consume fewer calories and lose weight.

Disease Prevention -

The body's ability to prevent and overcome various diseases through diet and exercise is truly astonishing. The fact that both Intermittent Fasting and veganism encourage and promote a balanced lifestyle consisting of healthy disease-fighting foods and regular physical activity makes them both conducive to disease prevention.

On one hand, IF claims to reduce the risk of cancer and various neurological disorders, while on the other hand, veganism claims to be the best approach for the prevention of heart disease and other chronic diseases. The approaches of these lifestyles and the types of diseases they benefit may differ, but their focus on health promotion is undoubtedly the same across the board.

Simplified Lifestyle -

Intermittent Fasting and veganism may sound complicated enough on their own, but combining these lifestyles can actually simplify your life more than you think. The fasting schedule will conveniently dictate when you eat, and the vegan diet will lay out what you eat at those pre-planned meal times, making the rest fall into place almost effortlessly.

Human nature has a way of overcomplicating even the simplest of things, so don't let your diet and lifestyle be the victim of this tendency. Sure, it may take a few weeks of trial and error to figure out what works best for you, but it won't be long before you start reaping some significant benefits.

Differences

The fundamental principles of Intermittent Fasting and veganism certainly overlap substantially, but a few obvious differences exist as well. In some cases, these differences are minor and perhaps insignificant, but there are a few specific cases in which these lifestyles seem to stand at polar opposites.

Dietary Conditions -

Intermittent Fasting was first popularized by muscular men in the fitness industry who were basically living on chicken breasts, raw egg whites, and whey protein shakes. Veganism, on the other hand, was built on the belief that humans should not consume any food that comes from animal sources in order to prevent the exploitation of these beings. Over the years, this concern for animals has extended to include the health and environmental benefits of a plant-based diet as well.

The main difference in the dietary conditions between these two lifestyles comes about in the discussion of protein, precisely the effect of animal protein versus plant protein. Many people in the IF community believe that a high-protein diet consisting mainly of animal products gives the best results, while the vegan community as a whole advocate for a diet rich in plant protein, healthy fats, and complex carbohydrates. As such, you'll sometimes hear people say that you can be a vegan intermittent faster, but you can't be an intermittent fasting vegan.

Carbohydrate Intake -

Taking the discussion of dietary conditions one step further, the topic of carbohydrates is of particular importance in the worlds of Intermittent Fasting and veganism.

Eating a high-carb diet while fasting can be counterproductive due to the relationship between carbohydrates and blood sugar. When you ingest carbs, your body breaks it down into sugar, and your blood sugar levels rise, increasing your insulin levels. As we know, an increase in insulin can lead to undesirable weight gain.

A vegan diet, however, is naturally reasonably high in carbohydrates, and this can be difficult to avoid. Even if you eat a high-protein, high-fat vegan diet with plant-based protein sources such as quinoa, chickpeas, lentils, Ezekiel bread, and vegetables don't go without some added carbohydrates too.

Availability of Information -

The term Intermittent Fasting has only been around since 2006 while the term vegan was coined back in 1944, making veganism a much more researched and scientifically advanced practice.

Opinions are, of course, always changing, especially with the diet mentality that continues to plague our society today, but the vegan diet is certainly more understood regarding long-term benefits and potential risks. There are even individuals on this earth who have been fully vegan for life. Apart from the research side things, there are also just more sources out there to learn about the vegan diet in general. From cookbooks and blog posts to podcasts and personal experience, the information that is available to the public makes it easier for potential vegans to make an educated and informed decision.

The Compound Concerns

Just as Intermittent Fasting and veganism provide tremendous benefits both on their own and together, they also raise some concerns. A lifestyle which includes both fasting and a vegan diet means that you have to take extra precautions to ensure that you are getting enough macronutrients and micronutrients from the foods you are eating.

It also means that you now not only need to think about the foods which you are consuming, but also the times in which you are consuming them. This may feel somewhat like a puzzle at the start, but with a little bit of experimentation, the pieces should fit together soon enough.

Digestive Problems -

Any change in diet or lifestyle, no matter how big or small, can lead to a number of digestion issues. Even if you are implementing IF on an already vegan diet, you may still experience symptoms such as constipation, diarrhea, and bloating.

Since the bacteria in your gut is optimized for the types of foods you usually eat, a simple shift such as going from high-carb, low-fat to high-fat, high-protein could wreak havoc on your digestive system. By changing your eating patterns slowly over time, you may be able to alleviate some of this gastrointestinal distress.

Social Limitations -

Being vegan in a predominantly meat-eating world can be stressful enough as it is, especially when it comes to social situations. Add Intermittent Fasting to that, and you now have a whole other factor in the equation that you need to solve.

Say you're making brunch plans with friends. You're probably used to checking the menu for vegan options, but now you also need to agree on a time that fits within your eating window.

Then, of course, there are those individuals who just don't understand why you lead the lifestyle that you do, which can result in them mocking and ridiculing you. These two things combined can be both frustrating and exhausting, making social situations a cause of stress rather than a form of enjoyment.

Overall Health -

Following a vegan diet means that you need to be extra mindful of the things you are putting into your body to ensure that you are not deficient in any nutrients or vitamins. For example, most doctors agree that all vegans should be supplementing B12 since it is just not possible to fulfill its need on a plant-based diet.

Being deficient in vitamins or minerals can lead to health problems such as bad skin, brittle hair and nails, low energy, muscle cramps, brain fog, and poor sleep. Since many of these symptoms are the same ones that can occur in connection with Intermittent Fasting as well, you want to be careful not to further worsen the effects.

Despite these apparent contradictions at times, there are ways to make such dissimilarities work for you and your lifestyle. After all, the appeal of both Intermittent Fasting and veganism lies in the flexibility that these ways of eating allow.

Intermittent Fasting & Keto Diet

Many health-conscious people around the world combine Intermittent Fasting and keto diet to drop weight and keep certain health conditions in check.

While both have solid research backing their claimed benefits, many people still wonder if it is safe and effective to combine the two.

Well, in my opinion, it is. Let me explain why.

What is the Keto Diet?

The ketogenic (keto) diet is something that has come up a fair amount of times in this book. The keto diet is a high-fat, yet extremely low-carb way of eating.

Carbohydrate intake is typically reduced to under 50 grams per day, thereby forcing your body to rely on fats, instead of glucose, as its primary energy source.

When you follow a keto diet, your body goes into the phase of ketosis. In this metabolic state, your body breaks down fats to form water-soluble biomolecules called ketone bodies to serve as an alternative source of fuel.

Since this diet burns the unwanted fat pockets, it is an effective way to shed pounds. But, apart from that, it has several other advantages as well.

The keto diet has been successfully used for nearly a century to treat epilepsy and has also demonstrated promising results for other neurological disorders.

For example, the keto diet may improve the mental symptoms in people with Alzheimer's disease.

What's more, it may also improve insulin resistance, reduce blood sugar, and lower heart disease risk factors such as triglyceride levels.

Potential Benefits of Fasting While on the Keto Diet

If you practice Intermittent Fasting while still following the ketogenic diet, it could offer the following benefits:

Triggering ketosis sooner

Remember the process of ketosis I told you about in Fat Fasting. The easiest way to trigger ketosis is to reduce your carbohydrate consumption.

Keto diet involves very low carb intake to force your body to go into ketosis. Many IF diets also tell you eat less carbs. This means, with Intermittent Fasting, you are already depriving yourself of carbohydrates and glucose, thus mimicking the actual process that takes place in a keto diet. Therefore, if your goal is to get into ketosis, IF can help you reach ketosis even faster.

At the same time, the keto diet also makes Intermittent Fasting more doable since it adapts your body to work with ketones. In addition, most people naturally eat less on keto due to the high satiety level, which means they are already used to fasting.

Avoiding the side effects of ketosis

Intermittent Fasting can prevent some common uncomfortable side effects, like the keto flu. (Another way to reduce the side effects associated with keto diet is by taking exogenous ketones!)

Keto can make your fasting periods more manageable. For example, if you eat a diet rich in carbs, you may find it challenging to practice IF as the body continually switches between glucose and ketones for fuel. By continuing a keto diet even during feeding periods, your body will keep running on ketones continuously, and not worry about glucose availability.

More Fat Loss

One of the biggest reasons people start Intermittent Fasting is to lose weight.

Being in ketosis reduces appetite and increases satiety levels, thus making it much easier to do Intermittent Fasting.

During IF, your daily calorie intake is already restricted, thus helping you to control your weight.

Also, the smaller eating windows eliminate unnecessary snacking, especially late at night.

And while you are eating all of that healthy fat, your body continues to break down the extra stored fat in your body to be used as energy—both while you are actually fasting and "fasting" with fats via the keto diet.

Controls blood sugar levels

During IF, since the body has to alternate between availability and non-availability of glucose, it can lead to spikes in blood sugar, causing brain fog, low energy, mood swings, and other side effects.

But if you're on a ketogenic diet, your body will stay in ketosis and not depend on glucose. This will keep your blood sugar stabilized.

Increasing the self-healing power of the body

As we know, Intermittent Fasting activates autophagy in the body cells and thus helps to recycle damaged proteins and remove harmful and toxic compounds from the body.

Different processes of autophagy are triggered when two things occur:

- The body is starved
- Protein and carbohydrates are restricted

Both of these happen, when you implement Intermittent Fasting on your ketogenic diet. Therefore, by combining the two, you can reap the benefits of autophagy in an efficient and healthy way.

Tips to Carry Out Fasting on Keto

So, if you're ready to combine Intermittent Fasting with your ketogenic diet, then here are my tips for success:

Ensure that you still eat enough

Due to Intermittent Fasting, you will naturally eat less, but make sure you eat nutritious ketogenic foods to avoid any nutrient deficiencies or metabolic issues.

You may even use a website or app to calculate the ideal caloric intake and the ketogenic macros for each day, and then track them to be sure you are getting sufficient nutrition.

Track your ketones

Although fasting can really help to stay in ketosis, it is still crucial to make sure you aren't eating too many carbohydrates or doing something else to kick you out of ketosis. Measure your ketone levels often to make sure you are actually in ketosis!

So Should You Combine Them?

Combining ketogenic diet and Intermittent Fasting is likely to be safe for most people.

- However, women who are pregnant or breastfeeding, and those with a history of eating disorders must avoid IF.
- People who have certain health issues, such as heart disease or diabetes, should consult their healthcare provider first before trying Intermittent Fasting on their ketogenic diet.
- Some people may find that fasting while on the keto diet is too difficult, or they may experience some adverse reactions, such as irritability and fatigue, and overeating on non-fasting days.

Therefore, even though some people may get successful results by merging Intermittent Fasting and keto diet, it is essential to note that combining both of them might not work for everyone.

Always remember that Intermittent Fasting is not compulsory to reach ketosis and see success with the keto diet, even though it can be used as a useful tool to do so quickly.

Keto diet is a broad topic. So, if you are interested to know about it more and maybe eventually practice both Intermittent Fasting and ketogenic diet together for becoming fit and healthier, then don't forget to check out my book on Ketogenic Diet.

Conclusion

Intermittent Fasting will provide you with a ton of great benefits and can help you lose weight while not feeling deprived in the process. And with the different methods that are available with IF, it is something you will really enjoy and will be able to fit into your daily schedule without much hassle.

Inside this guidebook, we looked at IF and how it can be so much more effective than your current eating plan. With the current fast food diets, we are taking in too many calories and getting into a horrible cycle that makes us sick. The body may crave those bad foods because they provide it with an easy and constant source of fuel, but we are slowly setting ourselves up for a whole bunch of chronic illnesses.

Intermittent Fasting helps us to change all of that. It gives us the option to cut down on the unnecessary calories we consume during the day while also naturally speeding up the metabolism.

To add to that during your fasting schedule, you will not give the body a constant source of glucose any longer, so it must rely on stored glycogen and other resources. Thus, it is no wonder that IF can help solve health problems while also helping you to lose weight.

My main objective with this book was to provide you with all of the information you could ever hope for on

Intermittent Fasting and how it affects the female form. And, now at the end of this guide, I am sure you have all the skills needed to not only get started on your own unique Intermittent Fasting journey but also be able to do so with confidence.

Some of the skills featured in the guide that I hope readers will find useful are:

- How to choose the right IF plan to meet your specific health goals
- How to plan or alter exercise routines to be the most effective throughout your new fasting plan, from helping the body adjust in the first few weeks to making changes to your regular fitness routine based on how the body reacts to Intermittent Fasting
- How to stay focused and determined even through the hardest of days of an Intermittent Fasting lifestyle
- How and when are the best ways/times to make changes or alterations to a personalized IF plan

From here, the next step is to finish gathering your information and get your first Intermittent Fasting plan together!

Fasting can be complicated, but the more information you have, the better are your chances to succeed at short-term and long-term health goals. As you set up your fasting plan, remember that there is no major hurry to get started with Intermittent Fasting as it is meant to be employed as a lifestyle change, or primarily a lifelong practice that can be:

- Developed based on an individual's current health, wellness, dietary and fitness needs
- Adjusted based on health changes over the years
- Put on pause for necessary circumstances like pregnancy for women or any kind of illness that could be worsened, rather than helped, by Intermittent Fasting
- Picked up again without much frustration or concern when the participant is ready to do so

An Important Warning:

Intermittent Fasting can be complicated for people who have problems with blood sugar regulation, suffer from hypoglycemia, diabetes, etc. If you are part of any of these categories, it is recommended that you consult your doctor or nutritionist before adjusting your meal schedule. More care is needed for these particular cases, and therefore, it is recommended that you do what your healthcare provider suggests.

Tips To Succeed At Intermittent Fasting

Regardless of the type of Intermittent fasting method you choose, here are some essential tips to stay on track, maximize the benefits and make the entire process go more smoothly before, during and after your fast.

Consult a doctor to know if you are fit to start fasting:

Even though you are someone with a clean bill of health, it is crucial to alert your personal physician of your plans.

As a rule of thumb, if you are a pregnant or lactating woman, a kid under 18 years of age or are taking prescription drugs due to underlying medical problems, don't practice IF.

The ideal option for those who can't fast is to transition to cleaner eating, that is eliminating rich, fatty, sugary, or highly processed foods and consuming whole fruits, vegetables and whole grains in their most natural state.

Make sure your fast fits into your lifestyle:

Plan your fasting schedule in such a way that allows you to go out with your friends and family, and enjoy your free time and weekends.

Also, avoid fasting during high-stress events or times as that can cause excessive exertion.

Prepare yourself and your home:

Before fasting, make sure that you are emotionally prepared and well-rested.

Remind yourself about your health goals and the reason you are doing the fast.

Lastly, get your house in order. Scan your pantry and get rid of any tempting foods or beverages that are not aligned with your fasting goals.

Stay hydrated:

Drink enough water and non-calorie drinks like herbal teas each day while fasting.

Always take your multivitamin supplements:

Since you will be missing many of the vitamins and minerals when fasting, it is necessary to take supplements to get most or all of your vitamin needs.

You may also choose vitamins in liquid form for easier digestion, but the best bet is to consult a doctor who knows you the best or who can advise you on the matter.

Engage in fun distractions:

When you get bored during your fasting schedule, treat yourself to a massage or manicure-pedicure session.

You can also go to the mall and do some window shopping for the new clothes you'll be able to wear once you lose weight.

However, avoid hunger triggers like going out to dinner and watching your friends eat. Also, stay away from all those mouth-watering food photos on social media.

Take a little help:

For that extra push, convince your friend or partner to fast with you. If nobody agrees, then you can also check out online support groups.

In case none of those work, remember you are our best friend. Try journaling your thoughts or recording small videos on your phone.

Take rest:

Dodge strenuous activities on fasting days, although light exercises such as yoga, a short walk, light cardio can be beneficial.

Increase the taste:

Season meals liberally with garlic, herbs, spices or vinegar. These foods are much low in calories and yet full of flavor, which can help reduce feelings of hunger.

Choose nutrient-rich foods after fasting:

Eating foods rich in fiber, vitamins, minerals, and other nutrients help keep blood sugar levels stable and helps prevent nutrient deprivation. A balanced diet also contributes to weight loss and overall health.

Don't overeat before a fast:

This "last supper" mentality is a rookie mistake that will give you indigestion, a poor night's sleep, and will adversely affect your stomach and brain. You will also find it difficult to fast the next day.

Avoid overindulging in a final feast before the fast. Instead, include lean meat, healthy fats, and lots of vegetables in your meal. You can also add some fruits for some natural sugar.

Don't try to be a hero:

Listen to your body and if you ever feel you're pushing too hard or too far, take a break. Immediately stop fasting if there are symptoms such as weakness, dizziness, and heart palpitations.

Outlook

There are various ways to do Intermittent Fasting, and there is not a single plan that works for everyone. To get the best outcomes, you must try different styles to see what suits your lifestyle and preferences.

For the best outcomes, it is essential to eat a healthy and balanced diet on non-fasting days. If necessary, a person can seek expert help to personalize their intermittent fasting program and avoid pitfalls.

Are all kinds of intermittent fasting styles safe?

People have been practicing fasting for millennia, but their safety depends more on who is fasting than the style of fasting.

People who suffer from malabsorption, low blood sugar, or other illnesses should seek the advice of their health care provider.

While most people can safely practice many fasting styles, extreme types of intermittent fasting, such as the Warrior Diet, can result in inadequate intake of nutrients such as fiber, vitamins, and minerals. Therefore, people should approach these forms of fasting with caution.

Busting Common Intermittent Fasting Myths

Here are some of the misconceptions you need to dismantle before starting your Intermittent Fasting journey:

Your metabolism will slow down:

Some people think that since they are not regularly eating, their metabolic rate will slow down and they will gain weight.

However, the truth is, not eating for a few hours will not adversely affect your metabolism. In fact, as we have discussed, it will actually help you lose weight and become healthy.

You'll lose weight and become extremely fit if you do Intermittent Fasting:

Losing weight actually depends on your total calorie intake. If someone overeats during the refueling period, then they will find it difficult to lose weight.

Also, if you want to become fit, Intermittent Fasting alone won't help you. You will have to exercise as well.

You can eat as much as you want after you stop Intermittent fasting:

No, you still have to be careful about what you eat. If you eat unhealthy food items in your eating time, then Intermittent Fasting will not give you the desired results.

Hunger pangs are bad for you:

Hunger pains or hunger pangs are caused by strong stomach contractions when it is empty. According to research, hunger pains won't do you any harm, so you need not worry about them.

Exercise should not be done on an empty stomach:

This is another common misconception that you should not worry about. In fact, exercising on an empty stomach has significant health benefits.

You'll enjoy your meals less:

Many people think that they won't be able to enjoy their meals because of hunger, which will force them to eat fast.

But, in reality, the opposite happens. You start eating more mindfully and enjoy your meals a lot more since you know it would be a long time before you can eat again.

Questions About Intermittent Fasting

Is an Intermittent Fasting Diet the Right Choice For Me?

It is essential to realize that the key is nutrition and finding an approach that can work for you in the long-term. This is where an Intermittent Fasting plan is a particularly exciting option when compared to other dietary methods.

So does an IF diet produce results when compared to other diets? The answer to that is a huge, resounding yes. For example, using a 16-hour fast will keep your body in a fat burning state for most part of the day!

And, then when you have all your calories during a relatively small eating window, it stops your body from entering a starvation mode and desperately hanging onto body-fat.

Compared to a regular reduced-calorie diet, this is a huge difference. While any reduced-calorie method will initially lead to fat-loss, your body being an efficient machine will compensate by slowing down your metabolic activities (the exact opposite of what you'd want) and holding onto body fat.

Is an Intermittent Fasting diet restrictive?

Any fitness diet, by its very nature, involves making smart food choices. If someone tries to sell you the pancake diet, run a mile away! Eating rubbish can never be the right choice.

However, most diets will require you try to eat clean all the time. This is a very tough task to do and is directly linked to eating 12 doughnuts in one sitting after a few weeks of deprivation!

Even though Intermittent Fasting involves healthy food choices, it does give you some wiggle room. It is difficult to overeat junk food in a small eating window after you have already had healthy food. IF does let you eat enough to stop you from falling off the wagon, though.

Perhaps the real advantage of IF is that it can be adopted as a lifestyle rather than a quick, short-term approach. With most fitness diets, even if you do manage to follow them long enough to get results, they are usually followed by a rebound – that is, a return to fat gain and poor eating. Since Intermittent Fasting is a long-term solution, this problem effectively disappears.

Should I take vitamins when I intermittently fast?

It is more critical than ever to take vitamins and supplements when fasting, as you are skipping meals that were helping to supply you with those vital nutrients, and it's crucial that you replace them.

The biggest problem with vitamins and fasting is that taking a vitamin pill in a fasted state may result in stomach pain, nausea, and diarrhea. To avoid these unpleasant, unsettling effects, try and get your vitamins down while in the fed state. If this is impossible, try taking your vitamins at night so you can sleep through the discomfort.

Alternatively, you might choose vitamins in liquid form, as they are easier to digest while fasting. If you don't usually take vitamins, a basic multivitamin that provides 100% of your daily intake is a great start to ensure you are not missing out on anything while intermittently fasting.

Why would anyone fast who doesn't want to lose weight?

It may seem odd for anyone who has their weight under control to change their eating habits or patterns and consider Intermittently Fasting. After all, aren't they already living the dream?

But, let us not forget about all the other benefits of IF:

- **Fasting for busy people with poor eating habits:** People who travel a lot for business often end up feeling less energetic of the time, due to poor eating habits developed as a result of airport restaurants and late-night vending machines.
- **Fasting for health benefits:** Some people swear by fasting because they feel it improves their sleep, mental clarity, and helps them control and maintain chronic diseases such as diabetes, cardiovascular disease, multiple sclerosis, fibromyalgia, chronic fatigue syndrome, cancer and the side effects from chemotherapy.
- **Fasting for athletes:** Fasting offers a consistent method of fueling and resting the body that works under many of the same principles as training and rest days. Thus it offers athletes a much more convenient way to

ensure that they consume the food they need to train than the other option of eating small meals every 2 or 3 hours. It also allows them to maintain a nutrition routine that provides a lengthier feeding time, which can be enjoyed with friends and family.

Why do I get headaches when I fast and how can I stop them?

Complaints of headaches, especially when beginning an IF program, are quite common.

If you are waking with a headache, you may not have hydrated yourself enough the night before. Not drinking plenty of water is one of the biggest culprits behind headaches during fasting, and thus drinking water should be imbibed throughout the fasting/feeding process.

Headaches can also be one of the side effects of the detoxifying process that occurs in Intermittent Fasting and will be especially prevalent in the beginning stages of incorporating the program into your health regime.

Is Intermittent Fasting safe for women?

Women are more hormonally sensitive than men. Because of this, they may respond more intensely to the challenges of Intermittent Fasting. They need to consult a medical professional before starting an IF program, especially if they have menstrual and fertility issues.

Once Intermittent Fasting has been undertaken, women should also pay special attention to their menstrual cycle, and seek medical guidance if they begin missing periods.

If you experience hormonal sensitivity, try the Crescendo method of fasting. It is a modified technique of IF that helps the female body adapt to fasting.

- Fast for 12-16 hours
- On fasting days, stick to light workouts such as yoga or light cardio
- Fast on 2-3 nonconsecutive days per week
- After a few weeks, add another day of fasting and monitor how it goes.
- Drink loads of water
- Save strength training for feeding periods or feeding days

Why can't I have a protein shake when I'm fasting?

You can't eat food when you are intermittently fasting – hence you can't drink a protein shake. People get confused about protein shakes. Check out diet, fitness, and nutrition and health websites if you don't believe me. I shake my head in wonder every time I see this question asked.

If you are on a 5:2 type of Intermittent Fasting program and you are consuming 500 to 600 calories on your "low" days, feel free to indulge in one or 2 of these shakes if they don't bring you over your total calorie count. If you are on whole day fasting or in the fasting portion of your time restricted IF cycle such as 16:8, don't even think about it!

How can I fast when I'm on vacation?

Try 5:2 Intermittent Fasting. Because you are confining your fasting to 2 non-consecutive days of the week, you can automatically end up with a 4-day feeding period. This will allow you to enjoy and eat during holidays and vacations.

To Summarize Everything

Intermittent Fasting can have some very positive benefits for someone trying to lose weight or increase lean body mass. Men and women tend to have different results. And the only way to find out is by experimenting. There are several ways to execute Intermittent Fasting:

Casual fasting: Probably the easiest method for the person who wants to do the least amount of work. It is merely skipping a meal when convenient.

Fast and feed regularly: Fast for a certain number of hours, then consume all the calories within a period.

Eat normally, then fast 1 or 2 times a week: Eat your regular meals every day, then, take one or two days of the week in which you fast for 24 hours. For example, eat the last meal on Sunday night, and then do not eat until dinner the next day.

Remember: One of the rules of rebellion is to question everything. If this seems like something you'd like to try, try it! If it seems crazy to you, ask yourself why you think it sounds crazy, and do your research and experimentation before condemning it.

Don't forget that the purpose of this guide is to provide information, practical steps to follow and advice on how to master the fundamentals of Intermittent Fasting based on research and experience collected and shared on the topic. It is not meant to be used as a medical reference or as a sole source of IF knowledge, particularly for those with existing health conditions that could be affected by what and how much they are or are not eating on a daily basis.

Doing your own research is not only a good idea, but a critical first step in achieving success with any kind of major health plans, diets, or fitness routines, including Intermittent Fasting.

So, that completes the fundamentals of Intermittent Fasting for Women!

Now that you've learned the basics about IF, what it is and how it works, I sincerely hope that you'll be able to use it as a valuable support tool and regular lifestyle practice. I believe, from the bottom of my heart, that IF will not only help you to take control of your personal health but will also enable you to stay fit throughout the course of your life and become a healthier, happier version of yourself!

So, go, make your personalized plan and take your first steps toward a healthy lifestyle supported by Intermittent Fasting.

Resources Page

- Potential Benefits and Harms of Intermittent Energy Restriction and Intermittent Fasting Amongst Obese, Overweight and Normal Weight Subjects—A Narrative Review of Human and Animal Evidence. (2017, March 1). Retrieved June 20, 2019, from https://www.ncbi.nlm.nih.gov/pmc/articles/PMC5371748/
- Fasting for weight loss: an effective strategy or latest dieting trend? - PubMed - NCBI. (n.d.). Retrieved June 20, 2019, from https://www.ncbi.nlm.nih.gov/pubmed/25540982
- INTERMITTENT FASTING AND HUMAN METABOLIC HEALTH. (2015, August 1). Retrieved June 20, 2019, from https://www.ncbi.nlm.nih.gov/pmc/articles/PMC4516560/
- Is Intermittent Fasting Healthy or Just a Fad Diet? (2019, April 22). Retrieved June 20, 2019, from https://rightasrain.uwmedicine.org/body/food/is-intermittent-fasting-healthy
- Influence of short-term repeated fasting on the longevity of female (NZB x NZW)F1 mice. - PubMed - NCBI. (n.d.). Retrieved June 20, 2019, from

https://www.ncbi.nlm.nih.gov/pubmed/1085462 9
- Effects of intermittent feeding upon growth and life span in rats. - PubMed - NCBI. (n.d.). Retrieved June 20, 2019, from https://www.ncbi.nlm.nih.gov/pubmed/7117847
- The effects of intermittent or continuous energy restriction on weight loss and metabolic disease risk markers: a randomized trial in young overwei... - PubMed - NCBI. (n.d.). Retrieved June 20, 2019, from https://www.ncbi.nlm.nih.gov/pubmed/20921964/
- Usefulness of routine periodic fasting to lower risk of coronary artery disease in patients undergoing coronary angiography. - PubMed - NCBI. (n.d.). Retrieved June 20, 2019, from https://www.ncbi.nlm.nih.gov/pubmed/18805103
- Martin, B., Mattson, M. P., & Maudsley, S. (2006). Caloric restriction and intermittent fasting: Two potential diets for successful brain aging. Ageing Research Reviews, 5(3), 332–353. https://doi.org/10.1016/j.arr.2006.04.002
- Intermittent fasting vs daily calorie restriction for type 2 diabetes prevention: a review of human findings. - PubMed - NCBI.

(n.d.). Retrieved June 20, 2019, from https://www.ncbi.nlm.nih.gov/pubmed/24993615

- The Washington Post. (n.d.). Retrieved June 20, 2019, from https://www.washingtonpost.com/gdpr-consent/?destination=%2fnational%2fhealth-science%2ffasting-may-protect-against-disease-some-say-it-may-even-be-good-for- HYPERLINK "https://www.washingtonpost.com/gdpr-consent/?destination=%2fnational%2fhealth-science%2ffasting-may-protect-against-disease-some-say-it-may-even-be-good-for-the-brain%2f2012%2f12%2f24%2fe521ee8-3588-11e2-bb9b-288a310849ee_story.html%3fnoredirect%3don&noredirect=on"the-brain%2f2012%2f12%2f24%2fe521ee8-3588-11e2-bb9b-288a310849ee_story.html%3fnoredirect%3don HYPERLINK "https://www.washingtonpost.com/gdpr-consent/?destination=%2fnational%2fhealth-science%2ffasting-may-protect-against-disease-some-say-it-may-even-be-good-for-the-brain%2f2012%2f12%2f24%2fe521ee8-3588-11e2-bb9b-288a310849ee_story.html%3fnoredirect%3don&

noredirect=on"& HYPERLINK "https://www.washingtonpost.com/gdpr-consent/?destination=%2fnational%2fhealth-science%2ffasting-may-protect-against-disease-some-say-it-may-even-be-good-for-the-brain%2f2012%2f12%2f24%2f6e521ee8-3588-11e2-bb9b-288a310849ee_story.html%3fnoredirect%3don&noredirect=on"noredirect=on

- Cheng, C.-W., Villani, V., Buono, R., Wei, M., Kumar, S., Yilmaz, O. H., … Longo, V. D. (2017). Fasting-Mimicking Diet Promotes Ngn3-Driven β-Cell Regeneration to Reverse Diabetes. Cell, 168(5), 775-788.e12. https://doi.org/10.1016/j.cell.2017.01.040

- Cheng, C.-W., Adams, G. B., Perin, L., Wei, M., Zhou, X., Lam, B. S., … Longo, V. D. (2014). Prolonged Fasting Reduces IGF-1/PKA to Promote Hematopoietic-Stem-Cell-Based Regeneration and Reverse Immunosuppression. Cell Stem Cell, 14(6), 810–823. https://doi.org/10.1016/j.stem.2014.04.014

- Intermittent fasting during Ramadan attenuates proinflammatory cytokines and immune cells in healthy subjects. - PubMed - NCBI. (n.d.). Retrieved June 20, 2019, from https://www.ncbi.nlm.nih.gov/pubmed/23244540

- Usefulness of Routine Periodic Fasting to Lower Risk of Coronary Artery Disease among Patients Undergoing Coronary Angiography. (2008, October 1). Retrieved June 20, 2019, from https://www.ncbi.nlm.nih.gov/pmc/articles/PMC2572991/
- Autophagy, Metabolism, and Cancer. - PubMed - NCBI. (n.d.). Retrieved June 20, 2019, from https://www.ncbi.nlm.nih.gov/pubmed/26567363
- Essential role for autophagy in life span extension. - PubMed - NCBI. (n.d.). Retrieved June 20, 2019, from https://www.ncbi.nlm.nih.gov/pubmed/25654554
- Autophagy has a key role in the pathophysiology of schizophrenia. - PubMed - NCBI. (n.d.). Retrieved June 20, 2019, from https://www.ncbi.nlm.nih.gov/pubmed/24365867
- Therapeutic targeting of autophagy in neurodegenerative and infectious diseases. - PubMed - NCBI. (n.d.). Retrieved June 20, 2019, from https://www.ncbi.nlm.nih.gov/pubmed/26101267

- Short-term fasting induces profound neuronal autophagy. (2010, August 16). Retrieved June 20, 2019, from https://www.ncbi.nlm.nih.gov/pmc/articles/PMC3106288/
- Immunologic manifestations of autophagy. - PubMed - NCBI. (n.d.). Retrieved June 20, 2019, from https://www.ncbi.nlm.nih.gov/pubmed/25654553
- Exercise induces autophagy in peripheral tissues and in the brain. - PubMed - NCBI. (n.d.). Retrieved June 20, 2019, from https://www.ncbi.nlm.nih.gov/pubmed/22892563
- Caloric Restriction Mimetics Enhance Anticancer Immunosurveillance. - PubMed - NCBI. (n.d.). Retrieved June 20, 2019, from https://www.ncbi.nlm.nih.gov/pubmed/27411589
- Ketosis may promote brain macroautophagy by activating Sirt1 and hypoxia-inducible factor-1. - PubMed - NCBI. (n.d.). Retrieved June 20, 2019, from https://www.ncbi.nlm.nih.gov/pubmed/26306884
- Circadian autophagy rhythm: a link between clock and metabolism? (2012, July 1).

Retrieved June 20, 2019, from https://www.ncbi.nlm.nih.gov/pmc/articles/PMC3389582/
- Five-day fasting diet could fight disease, slow aging. (2017, July 26). Retrieved June 20, 2019, from https://www.sciencemag.org/news/2017/02/five-day-fasting-diet-could-fight-disease-slow-aging
- Michael Mosley answers questions about intermittent fasting. (2017, February 8). Retrieved June 20, 2019, from https://thefastdiet.co.uk/michael-answers-frequently-asked-questions/
- The Fast Diet: What To Know | US News Best Diets. (n.d.). Retrieved June 20, 2019, from https://health.usnews.com/best-diet/fast-diet
- The Fast Diet: Health & Nutrition | US News Best Diets. (n.d.). Retrieved June 20, 2019, from https://health.usnews.com/best-diet/fast-diet/health-and-nutrition
- Alternate day fasting for weight loss in normal weight and overweight subjects: a randomized controlled trial. (891, December 14). Retrieved June 20, 2019, from https://nutritionj.biomedcentral.com/articles/10.1186/1475-2891-12-146

- Alternate day fasting and endurance exercise combine to reduce body weight and favorably alter plasma lipids in obese humans. - PubMed - NCBI. (n.d.). Retrieved June 20, 2019, from https://www.ncbi.nlm.nih.gov/pubmed/23408502
- Alternate day calorie restriction improves clinical findings and reduces markers of oxidative stress and inflammation in overweight adults with mod... - PubMed - NCBI. (n.d.). Retrieved June 20, 2019, from https://www.ncbi.nlm.nih.gov/pubmed/17291990
- The effect on health of alternate day calorie restriction: eating less and more than needed on alternate days prolongs life. - PubMed - NCBI. (n.d.). Retrieved June 20, 2019, from https://www.ncbi.nlm.nih.gov/pubmed/16529878/
- Varady, K. A., & Hellerstein, M. K. (2007). Alternate-day fasting and chronic disease prevention: a review of human and animal trials. The American Journal of Clinical Nutrition, 86(1), 7–13. https://doi.org/10.1093/ajcn/86.1.7

- What Is the Warrior Diet and Is It Right for Me? (2019, April 9). Retrieved June 20, 2019, from https://aaptiv.com/magazine/warrior-diet
- Ketogenic Diet - StatPearls - NCBI Bookshelf. (2019, March 21). Retrieved June 20, 2019, from https://www.ncbi.nlm.nih.gov/books/NBK499830/
- A review of low-carbohydrate ketogenic diets. - PubMed - NCBI. (n.d.). Retrieved June 20, 2019, from https://www.ncbi.nlm.nih.gov/pubmed/14525681

Made in the USA
Middletown, DE
11 September 2019